AF577338

Specific Heart Muscle Disease

Specific Heart Muscle Disease

Edited by **Cecil Symons** MD FRCP

Consultant Physician and
Cardiologist
Royal Free Hospital
London

Tom Evans MB ChB FRCP FACC

Consultant Cardiologist
Royal Free Hospital
London

and **Andrew G Mitchell** BA BM BCh MRCP

Senior Registrar in Cardiology
Harefield and
Royal Free Hospitals,
London

with a Foreword by
W Proctor Harvey

Director of the Division
of Cardiology
Georgetown University Hospital
Washington, DC

WRIGHT · PSG
Bristol London Boston
1983

Published by
John Wright & Sons Ltd., 823–825 Bath Road, Bristol BS4 5NU, England.
John Wright PSG Inc., 545 Great Road, Littleton,
Massachusetts 01460, U.S.A.

British Library Cataloguing in Publication Data

Specific heart muscle disease.
1. Heart—Muscle—Diseases
I. Symons, Cecil II. Evans, Tom
III. Mitchell, Andrew G.
616.1'24 RC681.A3

ISBN 0 7236 0641 2

Library of Congress Catalog Card Number: 82-63049

Typeset and printed in Great Britain by
John Wright & Sons (Printing) Ltd. at The Stonebridge Press,
Bristol BS4 5NU

Preface

Much has been written about ischaemic heart disease and the cardiomyopathies. There are many syndromes in which cardiac disease may be an integral part of the overall clinical picture—these comprise the specific heart muscle disorders.

This book has been written in an attempt to cover the major syndromes in which heart muscle disease is an intrinsic part of another clinical syndrome. Frequently the heart muscle disease is extremely important in its own right and may contribute to either the diagnosis or even determine the prognosis of the patient. Professor Goodwin, in the opening chapter, sets the scene with an appraisal of the cardiomyopathies in general and shows how they are related to the various forms of specific heart muscle disease. Following on, each chapter deals with the consideration of the many different manifestations of disease by authors who have special experience of their subjects and who may have many cases of the problem under their own clinical care. Their presentations may, therefore, be much more personalized than are found in a textbook of medicine or cardiology. However, we believe that this can only be advantageous, especially where the subject under consideration occurs but rarely. It is hoped that the text covers the specialties and will be of interest to general physicians and cardiologists alike. We believe that many of the subjects have not been discussed in such a monograph in such depth before and that the reader will find the book valuable, as a source of information and reference.

C.S.
T.E.
A.G.M.

Contributors

Margaret E Billingham MD FACC
Professor of Pathology and Cardiac Pathologist, Stanford University School of Medicine and Medical Center, Stanford, California

Michael R Bristow MD PhD
Physician Specialist in Medicine, Cardiology Division, Stanford University Medical Center, Stanford, California

Tom Evans MB ChB FRCP FACC
Consultant Cardiologist, Royal Free Hospital, London

Hugh A Fleming MD FRCP
Consultant Cardiologist, Addenbrooke's Hospital and Regional Cardiac Unit, Papworth Hospital, Cambridge

John F Goodwin MD FRCP FACC
Professor of Clinical Cardiology, Royal Postgraduate Medical School; Consultant Physician, Hammersmith Hospital, London

John S Jenkins MD FRCP
Professor of Clinical Endocrinology, St. George's Hospital Medical School; Consultant Physician, St. George's Hospital, London

Andrew G Mitchell BA BM BCh MRCP
Senior Registrar in Cardiology, Harefield and Royal Free Hospitals, London

Celia M Oakley MD FRCP FACC
Consultant Cardiologist, Hammersmith Hospital; Senior Lecturer in Medicine, Royal Postgraduate Medical School, London

Peter J Richardson MB BS MRCP
Senior Lecturer in Cardiology, King's College Hospital Medical School, London

Cecil Symons MD FRCP
Consultant Physician and Cardiologist, Royal Free Hospital, London

Michael M Webb-Peploe BA MB BChir FRCP
Consultant Physician and Cardiologist, St. Thomas' Hospital, London

Alex A Wodak MD FRACP MRCP
Research Fellow, Liver Unit, King's College Hospital, London

Contents

Foreword

It has been evident for a number of years that cardiomyopathies are much more commonplace than previously had been realized. Formerly considered rare diseases, it is now apparent that they are not uncommon. There are several reasons for this misconception in the past: in the first place, most physicians several decades ago clearly were not familiar with cardiomyopathies. In addition, they were often considered as an ill-defined group, described and classified by a number of terms: primary myocardial disease, myocarditis, myocardosis, myocardiopathy and many others. Because they were poorly recognized, as well as considered by many as uncommon, they were not carefully searched for. Therefore, they were overlooked and misdiagnosed. Since cardiomyopathies are often mimickers of other diseases, they therefore have been erroneously diagnosed as something else.

Even today, some are surprised at the prevalence of cardiomyopathies and tend to think of them as a new disease entity. Certainly this is not the case, but they are now better detected and correctly diagnosed.

Along with my colleagues here at Georgetown University Medical Center, I became interested and actively searched for cardiomyopathies about 35 years ago. My interest and awareness of cardiomyopathies was stimulated by two colleagues at the time, Dr. William C. Manion, Chief of Cardiac Pathology at the Armed Forces Institute of Pathology, and Dr. Thomas Mattingly, then Chief of Cardiology at Walter Reed Medical Center. I was a consultant in Cardiology at Walter Reed Medical Center and, through these physicians, I started to see and recognize these patients. The truth of the saying, 'You find what you look for' was quickly borne out. We then looked for and found increasing numbers of patients with cardiomyopathies at Georgetown University Medical Center, and it was not many years before we had evaluated several hundred patients, predominantly those now classified as dilated (congestive) cardiomyopathy. We classified our patients as idiopathic (aetiology unknown) and specific (aetiology known). The Report of the World Health Organisation and International Society and Federation of Cardiology (WHO/ISFC) Task Force on the definition and classification of cardiomyopathies (1980)[1] has reinforced this principle in the definition of cardiomyopathies as 'heart muscle disease of unknown cause', and specific heart muscle disease as 'heart muscle disease of known cause or associated with disease of other systems'.

It was apparent from analysis of our first several hundred patients that, regardless of whether idiopathic or specific aetiologies, the clinical features, symptoms and signs were strikingly similar. In addition, some that we characterized as unknown in aetiology became specific (known) when autopsy studies were performed. It is of interest that, at that time, physicians in other cities would say to me, 'You may have cardiomyopathies in Washington, D.C., but we don't see many cases in our city'. Subsequently, however, physicians who saw these patients in institutions in Washington and moved to other cities promptly found patients with cardiomyopathies. Concomitantly, physicians in other cities who had not recognized them before began to look for cardiomyopathies and, of course, found them.

The present classification of cardiomyopathies is a logical one: (1) hypertrophic (with or without obstruction); (2) dilated (congestive); and (3) restrictive/obliterative. This simple classification encompasses the unknown (idiopathic) group. There is extensive literature concerning hypertrophic cardiomyopathies, more than that of the dilated and the restrictive types. Then, there are the specific (or known) cardiomyopathies.

This book, *Specific Heart Muscle Disease*, has been a needed one. It is a solid attempt to help fill this need. It is a compilation of chapters devoted to this group and is an up-to-date synopsis not only of clinical and laboratory features, but also of management.

W. PROCTOR HARVEY
Director of the Division of Cardiology,
Georgetown University Hospital,
Washington, D.C.

[1] *Br. Heart J.* 1980; **44**, 672–673.

Chapter 1

Terminology of disorders of cardiac muscle

John F. Goodwin

INTRODUCTION

The term cardiomyopathy was used for many years in an imprecise and vague fashion to denote diseases of the myocardium and in such a wide sense as to be virtually meaningless, since all cardiac disorders eventually affect the myocardium in some way. However, by common consent the term has now come to be used to denote an unusual myocardial disorder, not due to common forms of heart disease such as occlusive coronary, rheumatic, hypertensive or congenital heart disease.

The recognition of the various types of cardiomyopathy, based on a detailed analysis of structure and function,[1–3] supported the contention of Segal et al.[4] that the majority of cardiomyopathies were of uncertain cause, rather than being due to a specific, albeit rare, pathological myocardial process. In order to avoid confusion and to concentrate on the problems of the cardiomyopathies of uncertain cause, it was decided to modify the definition of cardiomyopathy[1] and separate such 'primary' conditions from the 'secondary' cardiomyopathies.[5]

Thus, cardiomyopathy is now defined as 'heart muscle disease of unknown cause', while the former 'secondary' cardiomyopathies have been termed 'rare specific heart muscle diseases'.[5] The cardiomyopathies as thus defined may be subdivided, according to the functional and structural features, into three groups: (*a*) hypertrophic, (*b*) congestive (dilated) and (*c*) restrictive/obliterative.

Hypertrophic Cardiomyopathy

This condition, which is inherited, and previously known as hypertrophic obstructive cardiomyopathy (idiopathic hypertrophic subaortic

Table 1
Characteristics of the cardiomyopathies

	Ventricles								
Type	*Shape*	*Hypertrophy*	*Dilatation*	*Systolic volume*	*Diastolic volume*	*Systolic function*	*Diastolic function*	*Mitral regurgitation*	*Genetic aspects*
Hypertrophic	Slit: angulated	+ + +	O	↓	N	↑↑ Cavity elimination: gradients	Relaxation and filling abnormal	(+)	Hereditary factor
Congestive (dilated)	Globular	+	+ + +	↑↑	↑↑	↓↓↓	N or ↓	+	Familial case rare
Restrictive/obliterative	Irregular due to intracavity fibrosis	+	O or +	N or ↓	N or ↓	↑	Cavity restriction. Obliteration in late stages	+ +	None

stenosis), is characterized by massive, patchy hypertrophy of the ventricular muscle, notably of the septum. The shape of the cavity of the left ventricle is grossly abnormal, the normal ellipsoid configuration being replaced by a slit, with angulation in the mid-portion. Systolic volume is reduced, but diastolic volume is normal. The main fault lies in diastole, relaxation and filling of the left ventricle being grossly disordered. Systolic function is excellent until the late stages of the disease in the minority of patients. Systolic pressure gradients across the outflow tract of the left ventricle are common, but do not indicate true obstruction to outflow.[6,7]

Congestive (Dilated) Cardiomyopathy

This diagnosis probably covers a number of conditions, all of which eventually result via a final common path in congestive cardiac failure. Congestive cardiomyopathy is entirely different from hypertrophic cardiomyopathy. Dilatation of the ventricles is the main feature and, being a diffuse disease, it usually involves both ventricles. Occasionally the right ventricle alone may be affected.[8] Systolic pump function is extremely poor and the situation is exactly the opposite to that of hypertrophic cardiomyopathy. Although hypertrophy of the ventricles occurs to varying degrees in congestive (dilated) cardiomyopathy, it never approaches the extent seen in hypertrophic cardiomyopathy.

The term 'dilated' has been preferred[9] to 'congestive' because it is more descriptive and emphasizes the differences from hypertrophic cardiomyopathy. It is also now appropriate because diagnosis can often be made before overt congestive failure develops. It is convenient, however, because of familiarity of usage, to retain the term 'congestive'.

There is probably no single cause of congestive cardiomyopathy; a multifactorial aetiology is likely. Of the causes or associated conditions that have been postulated, such as systemic hypertension, pregnancy, alcohol, virus infections and disorder of immunity, the most likely is probably virus infection leading to an auto-immune cellular dysfunction.[10] The other conditions may act as 'conditioning' factors.

Restrictive/Obliterative Cardiomyopathy

This term is used to describe cardiomyopathy in which the haemodynamic fault is restriction of filling of the ventricles, such as that which occurs in constrictive pericarditis. The usual cause of restrictive/obliterative cardiomyopathy is endomyocardial fibrosis (EMF). This occurs in two forms: the tropical variety[11,12] without eosinophilia, and the temperate clime variety with eosinophilia described originally by Löffler. The pathology of the two types is identical[13] and it has been suggested that they are the same disease.[14] In the later stages the endomyocardial fibrosis obliterates the ventricular cavities, reducing their volume and further increasing the restriction to inflow. Eosinophilic heart disease is dealt with in detail in a later chapter.

Certain conditions are not easily classifiable as either cardiomyopathy or specific heart muscle disease. Amyloid, when it involves the heart alone, may well deserve the definition of cardiomyopathy but when other organs are involved it is more properly considered as a specific heart muscle disease. In other situations some pathological states are sufficiently well associated to be included as a specific heart muscle disease, e.g. alcoholic heart disease, peripartal heart disease, etc. There are in addition a number of entities which at present cannot be classified according to the three forms of cardiomyopathy—hypertrophic, congestive or restrictive. These conditions do not present evidence of diffuse myocardial disorders but may be due to localized myocardial damage of unknown cause. They are:

1. Arrhythmic cardiomyopathy: heart failure due to repetitive intractable ventricular arrhythmia. (Alcoholic heart disease, sarcoidosis and ischaemic heart disease must be excluded before a positive diagnosis of cardiomyopathy is made.)
2. Conduction disorders: heart block of congenital and inherited nature.
3. Long QT syndromes.
4. Prolapsing mitral valve syndromes.
5. Angina with angiographically normal major coronary arteries and evidence of myocardial dyskinesia or infarction.

'Ischaemic Cardiomyopathy'

This term has erroneously been applied to patients with severe widespread occlusive coronary artery disease who do not give a history of myocardial infarction or angina but present with heart failure and progressive cardiomegaly. Such patients differ from patients with congestive (dilated) cardiomyopathy in having marked ventricular dyskinesia, but clinically they are very difficult to differentiate. The term 'ischaemic cardiomyopathy', while tempting to use, is misleading. The cause of the myocardial disorder is severe widespread occlusive coronary artery disease and, therefore, the condition does not come within the definition of the cardiomyopathies.

It must be emphasized that all the cardiomyopathies, by definition, are associated with normal major coronary arteries. In fact, in both hypertrophic and congestive cardiomyopathies, the major arteries are remarkably smooth, regular and of wide calibre. However, instances occur in which the myocardial impairment appears out of proportion to the extent of coronary artery disease and as there is good reason to believe that coincidental atherosclerotic coronary disease can occur in association with congestive cardiomyopathy, a precise diagnosis in some cases may not be achieved.

Rare Specific Heart Muscle Diseases

The WHO/ISFC Task Force Report[9] gives a list which is reproduced below with some modifications. A more complete list, under the title of secondary cardiomyopathies, has been provided by Fowler.[15]

Infective:
- *Myocarditis*
- Viral
- Rickettsial
- Fungal
- Bacterial
- Protozoal
- Metazoal

Metabolic:
- *Endocrine*
- Thyrotoxicosis
- Myxoedema
- Adrenal cortical failure
- Phaeochromocytoma
- Acromegaly
- Diabetes
- *Infiltration and Storage Diseases*
- Haemochromatosis
- Mucopolysaccharidosis
- Refsum's disease
- Hurler's syndrome
- Hunter's syndrome
- Niemann–Pick disease
- Hand–Schüller–Christian disease
- Fabry–Anderson disease
- Morquio–Ulrich disease

Deficiency Disorders:
- Disturbances of potassium metabolism
- Magnesium deficiency
- Nutritional disorders
- Kwashiorkor
- Anaemia
- Beri-beri

Connective Tissue Disorders:
- Systemic lupus erythematosus
- Rheumatoid arthritis
- Polyarteritis nodosa
- Scleroderma
- Dermatomyositis

Granulomas and Neoplasms:
- Sarcoidosis
- Leukaemia
- Secondary neoplasms
- Carcinoid

Neuromuscular Disorders:
- Friedreich's ataxia
- Myotonica dystrophica
- Duchenne's muscular dystrophy
- Facioscapulohumoral dystrophy

Sensitivity and Toxic Reactions:
- Sulphonamides
- Penicillin
- Cobalt
- Antimony
- Hematine
- Alcohol
- Isoprenaline
- Adriamycin
- Irradiation

The majority of the specific heart muscle diseases produce ventricular dilatation resembling congestive cardiomyopathy. Exceptions include localized infiltrations which may cause abnormalities of rhythm; Friedreich's ataxia and glycogen storage disease, which cause a hypertrophic type with systolic gradients; and carcinoid heart disease which produces endocardial fibrosis with pulmonary and tricuspid valve stenosis.

Most of the specific heart muscle diseases will be covered elsewhere in this work, but peripartal heart disease, the connective tissue disorders, diabetic heart disease and the relationship of myocarditis to cardiomyopathy are dealt with in this chapter.

PERIPARTAL HEART DISEASE

This is a syndrome of cardiac failure during the latter part of pregnancy or in the puerperium without obvious cause and without other heart disease.[16] Heart failure associated with pregnancy has been recognized since the middle of the nineteenth century. Many reports have been published from diverse parts of the world since 1930.

The clinical and haemodynamic features are those of congestive cardiomyopathy and the occurrence in late pregnancy or the puerperium may be no more than fortuitous. In North America the disease is more common in black than white patients, in multiparous, older women and in the presence of twin pregnancy and toxaemia.[17] Benchimol et al.[18] suggested that the aetiology was not uniform but that there were probably three main groups: those due to toxaemia of pregnancy, those due to pre-existing hypertension and those due to myocarditis. Work in the past two decades has scarcely clarified the issue much further, but Brockington[19] suggested that rapid, transient hypertension in the puerperium might be responsible for congestive heart failure that would recur in subsequent pregnancies. Although complete recovery may occur, recurrence in further pregnancies is common and carries a bad prognosis, as does pregnancy in patients with residual cardiomegaly after the first episode.[20] The clinical picture is one of congestive cardiomyopathy: there are no distinguishing features. It is uncertain whether peripartal cardiomyopathy is a distinct entity, although the tendency to recurrence in subsequent pregnancies may suggest this. Virus infection occurring at a vulnerable time for the patient may possibly be an explanation. Peripartal cardiomyopathy can occur in the absence of any risk or conditioning factors such as hypertension, alcohol, malnutrition and toxaemia of pregnancy.

Recently an interesting form of post-partum cardiac failure has been described from Zaria, Northern Nigeria, by Sanderson et al.[21] The condition (PPCF) is due not to heart muscle disease, but to excessive body-heating and to consumption of salt. Severe congestive heart failure with cardiomegaly and massive oedema follows. It has been postulated[22] that the excessive heating of the body, which is part of the ritual of childbirth for Hausa women, causes a reduction in peripheral vascular resistance so that the blood pressure can only be maintained by an increase in cardiac output. This difficulty in raising the blood pressure gives rise to further problems in dealing with excessive sodium and water loads and tends to aggravate oedema. The cardiac dilatation produced by the volume overload may possibly cause myocardial damage but typically in these patients cardiac output is high and complete recovery occurs after delivery.

It seems likely therefore that these patients do not have true peripartal cardiomyopathy. Sanderson's hypothesis, however, has been challenged by Davidson,[23] who argues that the condition may be due to salt retention and relative hypertension.

DIABETIC HEART DISEASE

The major cardiac complications of diabetes mellitus are unquestionably atherosclerotic coronary heart disease and systemic hypertension. The occurrence of a form of heart muscle disease, specific to diabetes, has been questioned. Because of the frequency of disease of small arteries elsewhere, it has been tempting to suppose that the small intramural coronary arteries may be affected in diabetes, but the evidence for this is not very strong. Although occlusive changes have been found in over 40 per cent of an unselected random sample of necropsies,[24] similar lesions have been found in patients who were not diabetic. Furthermore, a later study of the intramural vessels in the free wall of the left ventricle in diabetics did not reveal any obstructive lesions.[25]

Experimental studies in dogs made diabetic with alloxan showed increased stiffness of the left ventricle due to accumulation of glycoprotein. Regan *et al.*[26] concluded that chronic diabetes mellitus could alter myocardial composition and function independent of any vascular effects.

Clinical studies by Ahmed et al.[27] showed abnormal ventricular function in the absence of angiographic disease of the major coronary arteries in diabetics. These workers suggest that glycoprotein increments occur early in diabetes mellitus and are associated with reduced diastolic compliance of the ventricle. This might explain the allegedly high mortality after myocardial infarction in diabetics. Echocardiographic studies of young diabetic patients by Sanderson et al.[28] revealed abnormalities of myocardial function in all but 6 of 23 patients. These workers attributed the abnormalities to disease of the small myocardial vessels but the changes could have been on the basis of the findings of Ahmed et al.[27]

The existence of a specific 'diabetic' myocardial disease remains uncertain but there is little doubt that patients with diabetes who have coronary artery disease tend to fare worse than patients with coronary artery disease who are not diabetic.

THE CONNECTIVE TISSUE DISORDERS

Systemic Lupus Erythematosus (SLE)

The most common cardiac complications of SLE are hypertension and pericarditis. Rarely there is involvement of the mitral valve (Libman-Sachs endocarditis) and sometimes the myocardium may be affected, perhaps in up to 40 per cent of cases.[15] The myocardial lesions consist of deposition of fibrinoid material in the septa between the myocardial cells.[29] There may be arteritis and occlusion of small arteries including those of the conducting system.[30] Brigden et al.[29] also reported scarring of the papillary muscles. Clinically the common cardiac presentation is of pericarditis with chest pain, fever, pericardial friction and signs of effusion in some cases. Constriction is rare but has been reported. Heart failure may be due to systemic hypertension, myocardial involvement or mitral regurgitation, or to a combination of all these factors. Infective endocarditis may be a complication and conduction defects can occur. The electrocardiogram commonly shows abnormal but non-specific changes and a frequent feature is ST segment elevation due to pericarditis. Bundle branch block and atrioventricular block are rare.

Rheumatoid Arthritis

Pericarditis with constriction is relatively common. With the reduced incidence of acute tuberculous pericarditis in the United Kingdom, rheumatoid arthritis has become one of the more frequent causes of constrictive pericarditis. In severe rheumatoid disease pericardial disease with effusion may remain unsuspected unless specifically looked for. Signs of cardiac tamponade may be absent if the effusion has accumulated slowly. Cardiomegaly on chest radiography and low voltage complexes in the electrocardiogram should suggest the diagnosis, which can be confirmed by echocardiography. The pathology of the myocardium may reveal rheumatoid nodules but often there is non-specific fibrosis. Valvar lesions are rare but occasionally aortic regurgitation and mitral regurgitation are present, presumably the result of rheumatoid changes in the valves.

Ankylosing Spondylitis and Reiter's Syndrome

Direct involvement of the myocardium usually takes the form of involvement of the conducting tissue. All grades of heart block are well recognized, usually in association with aortic regurgitation. The pathology of the aorta and aortic valve closely resembles that of syphilis. Pericarditis may occur in Reiter's syndrome.

Diffuse Systemic Sclerosis

This disease affects the heart in several ways: replacement of cardiac muscle by connective tissue, small vessel disease of the myocardium, conduction defects, systemic hypertension and right ventricular congestive heart failure due to severe pulmonary hypertension resulting from involvement of the pulmonary arterioles. Occasionally ventilatory difficulties result from massive involvement of the skin and the chest wall leading to cor pulmonale. Pericarditis can also occur.

Dermatomyositis

Dermatomyositis may produce oedema between myocardial fibres, sometimes with lymphocytic infiltration and necrosis. Occasionally calcification is present. The pericardium may be involved and heart failure can occur. Conduction defects have been reported.

Periarteritis Nodosa

The necrotizing arteritis and micro-aneurysm formation that are the pathological features of periarteritis nodosa may involve the major coronary arteries and can cause myocardial infarction. Patchy fibrosis of the myocardium is common and a restrictive haemodynamic picture has been reported.[1] Pericarditis with effusion is well recognized. The pericarditis may be non-specific or uraemic in nature. Severe systemic hypertension may cause left ventricular hypertrophy and failure.

The coronary artery lesions of periarteritis nodosa bear some resemblance to the muco-cutaneous lymph node syndrome (Kawasaki syndrome), which is an acute illness of infants and young children described from Japan.[31] There is fever, cervical lymph node swelling, cardiomegaly and ECG evidence of myocardial ischaemia or infarction. The main coronary arteries have a severe arteritis and develop diffuse irregular aneurysms. Complications and modes of death are similar to those occurring in occlusive atherosclerotic coronary artery disease.

THE RELATIONSHIP OF MYOCARDITIS TO CARDIOMYOPATHY

As will be seen, certain specific forms of myocarditis are grouped with the specific heart muscle diseases. Since coxsackie and other viruses that are known to affect the heart may be associated with the development of congestive cardiomyopathy it is convenient to consider their relationship within the framework of the cardiomyopathies.

Viral myocarditis is well documented in animals[32] and is known to occur in man, often accompanied by pericarditis. Proof of viral myocarditis is often inferential because recovery of virus or viral antibody from heart muscle is usually impracticable or inconclusive. Nevertheless, a reliable diagnosis of viral myocarditis can often be made clinically but its relationship to congestive cardiomyopathy is speculative. Anecdotal reports are available which suggest that virus myocarditis may lead to cardiomyopathy.[33,34] The relationship between congestive cardiomyopathy and virus infections has been strengthened by the finding of high blood levels of coxsackie B 1–4 titres in the blood of patients with a short history of the disease; endomyocardial biopsy, however, revealed no evidence of myocarditis.[35] Possible explanations for these findings might be:

1. Chance association.
2. Virus infection in an already vulnerable heart.
3. Acute or subacute myocarditis.
4. Virus infection disappearing without trace but leaving in its wake a progressive impairment of cellular immunity leading to persistent destruction of myocardial function resulting in congestive cardiomyopathy after a long latent period. This supposition is strengthened by the finding of Fowles et al.[36] of a disorder of cellular immunity in patients with congestive cardiomyopathy.

While not providing any proof of a viral aetiology for congestive cardiomyopathy these reports are of especial interest. Another possible connection between myocarditis and congestive cardiomyopathy was suggested by Mason et al.,[37] who described changes of myocarditis on endomyocardial biopsy in a small group of patients who developed congestive heart failure of unknown cause. The endomyocardial biopsy lesions resolved on treatment with immunosuppressive agents.

It appears likely that viral myocarditis may follow three different pathways:

1. Complete recovery (which is usual).
2. The rapid onset of congestive heart failure (as described by Mason et al.[37]).
3. Apparent complete recovery with the development of congestive cardiomyopathy after several years as a result of a progressive disorder of cellular immunity set up by the virus infection.

Another explanation would be that the virus had affected a heart already rendered vulnerable by immunological deficiency.

The relationship of myocarditis to cardiomyopathy is a highly speculative area and much further work is required to consolidate ground already won.

REFERENCES

1. Goodwin JF, Gordon H, Hollman A, Bishop MB. Clinical aspects of cardiomyopathy. *Br Med J* 1961; **1**: 69.
2. Goodwin JF. Congestive and hypertrophic cardiomyopathies: a decade of study. *Lancet* 1970; **1**: 731.
3. Goodwin JF. International lecture. Prospects and predictions for the cardiomyopathies. *Circulation* 1974; **50**: 210.
4. Segal JP, Harvey WP, Gurel T. Diagnosis and treatment of primary myocardial disease. *Circulation* 1965; **32**: 837.
5. Goodwin JF, Oakley CM. The cardiomyopathies. *Br Heart J* 1972; **34**: 545.
6. Criley JM, Lewis KB, White RI et al. Pressure gradients without obstruction. A new concept of 'hypertrophic sub-aortic stenosis'. *Circulation* 1965; **32**: 881.
7. Goodwin JF. An appreciation of hypertrophic cardiomyopathy. *Am J Med* 1980; **68**: 797.
8. Fitchett DH, Neto JA, Oakley CM, Goodwin JF. Hydralazine in the management of left ventricular failure. *Am J Cardiol* 1979; **44**: 303.
9. Report of the WHO/ISFC Task Force on the definition and classification of cardiomyopathy. *Br Heart J* 1980; **44**: 672.
10. Goodwin JF. Predictions for the cardiomyopathies. In: Yu PN, Goodwin JF, eds. *Progress in cardiology*, vol. 10. Philadelphia: Lea & Febiger. 1981: 175.
11. Davies JNP. Endocardial fibrosis in Africans. *East Afr Med J* 1948; **25**: 117.
12. Parry EHO. Endomyocardial fibrosis. In: Wolstenholm GEW, O'Connor M, eds. *Cardiomyopathies*. Ciba Foundation Symposium. London: Churchill, 1964: 322.
13. Brockington I, Olsen EGJ. Löffler's endocarditis and Davies endomyocardial fibrosis. *Am Heart J* 1973; **85**: 308.
14. Olsen EGJ, Spry CJF. The pathogenesis of Löffler's myocardial disease and its relationship to endomyocardial fibrosis. In: Yu PN, Goodwin JF, eds. *Progress in cardiology*, vol. 8. Philadelphia: Lea & Febiger, 1979: 281.

15. Fowler NO. The secondary cardiomyopathy. In: Fowler NO, ed. *Myocardial diseases*. New York: Grune & Stratton, 1973: 337.
16. Goodwin JF. Peripartal heart disease. *Clin Obstet Gynecol* 1975; **18**: 125.
17. Walsh JJ, Birch GE, Black HC, Ferrans VJ, Hibbs RG. Idiopathic cardiomyopathy of the puerperium (postpartal heart disease). *Circulation* 1965; **32**: 19.
18. Benchimol AB, Carneiro RD, Schlesinger P. Postpartum heart disease. *Br Heart J* 1959; **21**: 89.
19. Brockington IF. Postpartum hypertensive heart failure. *Am J Cardiol* 1971; **27**: 650.
20. Demakis JG, Rahimtoola SH, Sutton GC et al. Natural causes of peripartal cardiomyopathy. *Circulation* 1971; **44**: 1053.
21. Sanderson JE, Adesanya CO, Anjorim F, Parry EHO. Postpartum heart failure. Heart failure due to volume overload? *Am Heart J* 1979; **97**: 423.
22. Sanderson JE. Oedema and heart failure in the tropics. *Lancet* 1977; **2**: 1159.
23. Davidson NMcD. Tropical oedema and peripartum cardiac failure. *Lancet* 1978; **1**: 145. (Letter.)
24. Schwartz CJ, Mitchell JRA. Relation between myocardial lesions and coronary artery disease. *Br Heart J* 1962; **24**: 761.
25. Roberts WC. Coronary arteries in fatal acute myocardial infarction. *Circulation* 1972; **45**: 215.
26. Regan TJ, Ettinger PO, Khan MI et al. Altered myocardial function and metabolism in chronic diabetes mellitus without ischaemia in dogs. *Circ Res* 1974; **35**: 222.
27. Ahmed SS, Regan TJ, Jaferi GA, Narang RM. Preclinical reduction of left ventricular function in diabetes mellitus. *Am Heart J* 1975; **89**: 153.
28. Sanderson JE, Brown DJ, Rivellese A, Kohner E. Diabetic cardiomyopathy? An echocardiographic study of young diabetics. *Br Med J* 1978; **1**: 404.
29. Brigden W, Bywaters E, Lessoff, M, Ross I. The heart in systemic lupus erythematosus. *Br Heart J* 1960; **22**: 1.
30. James T, Rupe C, Manto R. Pathology of the cardiac conduction system in systemic lupus erythomatosis. *Ann Intern Med* 1965; **63**: 402.
31. Kato H, Koike S, Yamamoto M, Ito Y, Yano E. Coronary aneurysm in infants and young children with acute febrile mucocutaneous lymph node syndrome. *Paediatrics* 1975; **86**: 892.
32. Kawii C, Matsumori A, Kataura Y, Takatsu T. Viruses of the heart: viral myocarditis and cardiomyopathy. In: Yu PN, Goodwin JF, eds. *Progress in cardiology*, vol. 7. Philadelphia: Lea & Febiger, 1978: 141.
33. Somerville W. Postcarditic myocardiopathy. *Postgrad Med J* 1972; **48**: 746.
34. Obesekere I, Hermon Y. Ventricular aneurysm: an appraisal of diagnosis and surgical treatment. *Br Heart J* 1972; **34**: 821.
35. Cambridge G, MacArthur CGC, Waterson AP, Goodwin JF, Oakley CM. Antibodies to coxsackie B viruses in congestive cardiomyopathy. *Br Heart J* 1979; **41**: 692.
36. Fowles PP, Beiber CP, Stinson EB. Defective *in vitro* suppressor cell dysfunction in idiopathic congestive cardiomyopathy. *Circulation* 1979; **59**: 483.
37. Mason JW, Billingham ME, Ricci DR. Treatment of acute inflammatory myocarditis assisted by endomyocardial biopsy. *Am J Cardiol* 1980; **45**: 1037.

Chapter 2

Amyloid heart disease

Celia M. Oakley

INTRODUCTION

Amyloid is an abnormal fibrillar protein which can be deposited in almost any organ of the body. The name amyloid was coined by Virchow because amyloid gives a colour reaction to iodine which is similar to that given by starch although not identical with it. The structure of the amyloid fibril and the pattern of deposition of it in the body differs according to five major forms of the disease. These are:

1. Primary amyloidosis in which there is no other detectable disease and the plasma proteins are normal.
2. Amyloidosis associated with myeloma in which there is an abnormal monoclonal plasma globulin.
3. Secondary amyloidosis associated with chronic suppuration such as in osteomyelitis, chronic infection as in tuberculosis or other chronic disorders particularly rheumatoid arthritis.
4. Familial amyloidosis which occurs in neuropathic, cardiopathic and nephropathic forms and also in familial Mediterranean fever in which again the kidney is chiefly involved.
5. Senile amyloid which seems to be a degenerative accompaniment of increasing old age.

Cardiac involvement is common in primary amyloid and in amyloidosis associated with multiple myeloma. Amyloid may infiltrate the skin and mucous membranes, the tongue, peripheral nerves and gastrointestinal tract as well as the heart. Although the kidneys are often also involved there is usually no clinical abnormality. In primary amyloid the amyloid fibrils are thought to be derived from immunoglobulin light chains usually of the lambda type. The amyloidosis associated with multiple myeloma is usually similar and presumptively derived from the abnormal globulin. In patients presenting with amyloid heart disease the existence of an underlying paraprotein is often cryptic.

In secondary amyloidosis clinical cardiac abnormality is uncommon because the myocardial deposits are small rather than massive as in primary amyloid.

Amyloid is commonly found in the hearts of those dying in advanced old age. The amount of amyloid in these hearts is very much less than that found in cardiac amyloidosis and rarely associated with any typical clinical abnormality, although its presence and other degenerative changes in the elderly heart may contribute to the tendency to heart failure which occurs in the elderly, typically with little seeming provocation.

Amyloid material is deposited in and around the walls of capillaries and small arteries and veins. It has characteristic staining reactions but in primary amyloidosis the staining is often less typical than it is in secondary amyloidosis. For example, the iodine reaction may be negative in the autopsy room and lead to the diagnosis being missed. Histologically amyloid stains apple green with Congo red and gives a metachromatic reaction to methyl violet. Intravenous injection of Congo red was used as a diagnostic test for amyloidosis, the Congo red pigment being removed from the circulating plasma because of the physical affinity of the amyloid material for the dye. However, a positive test depends on a massive amount of amyloid being present, it being necessary for more than 60 per cent of the Congo red to disappear from the plasma for the test to be declared positive, and perhaps 80 per cent for certainty. Allergic reactions as well as false negatives in primary amyloidosis were common and the test is no longer used.

Heart disease is not usually recognized until there is massive infiltration of the heart. The time course of the process before symptoms develop is quite unknown but the inexorable deterioration following diagnosis is known only too well and most patients are dead within a year. The disorder is less rare than generally supposed, many cases being missed even though the clinical and haemodynamic findings are distinctive. A clinical diagnosis can usually be made provided the possibility is considered.

Amyloidosis of the heart is uncommon below the age of 40 and most patients are in late middle or old age. This contrasts with secondary amyloidosis which is usually seen in much younger people, is known to be reversible with complete clinical recovery, provided the predisposing cause can be removed, and in which loss of the amyloid from affected organs has been demonstrated.

PATHOLOGY

The heart is overweight and appears to show concentric hypertrophy of both ventricles. There is little enlargement as the ventricular cavities are not dilated. The heart is firm and rubbery in consistency so that it fails to collapse on the post mortem table. The general appearance may be not unlike that in hypertrophic cardiomyopathy with which it has been confused grossly.

Important pointers to the likelihood of amyloid may be petechiae on the outside of the heart, there may be a pericardial effusion associated with visible focal amyloid deposits in the pericardium and the cut surface may have a 'lardaceous' look.

The endocardium is involved in most patients but any valvar abnormality is usually slight. When mitral regurgitation occurs it is usually attributable to heavy infiltration of the papillary muscles. Occasionally thrombosis occurs over the irregular endocardium, predisposing to embolism.

Most of the amyloid is in the myocardium, its mass being responsible for the thickening of the walls of the ventricles and even the atria. Microscopically the amyloid is found between the myocardial fibres, parting and compressing them, as well as in the walls of the intramural coronary arteries and veins sometimes with compromise of the lumen. Amyloid deposits in the sino-atrial and atrio-ventricular nodes, as well as in the conducting bundles, explains the frequency of sino-atrial dysfunction and fascicular blocks on the ECG as well perhaps as the seemingly excessive sensitivity to digitalis.[1-4]

CLINICAL FEATURES

Primary amyloid usually presents with heart failure, with complaint of fatigue, shortness of breath or oedema and sometimes with angina.

Involvement of the conducting tissue, the low blood pressure and digitalis intoxication may all contribute to syncope which can be another presenting feature.[5]

Rarely the patient may present because of a rash. This is caused by bleeding in the skin where this is the seat of amyloid infiltration. Sometimes petechiae are profuse, particularly in the periorbital tissue and on the face and neck. The tongue may feel rubbery and it may be enlarged. Rarely enlargement of the tongue or blurring of speech is a presenting feature.

The patient feels and looks unwell, the skeletal muscles may be weak and rarely are enlarged on account of amyloid infiltration. The lymph nodes may be involved and enlarged and perineural deposition may be palpable and associated with a clinical mononeuritis. Involvement of the gastro-intestinal tract may lead either to diarrhoea or to constipation. The liver is usually enlarged in association with a high venous pressure although there may be no amyloid in it in the primary form.

The spleen is not usually palpable. The heart beat is usually regular although bradycardia is common either from sino-atrial disease or from digitalis intoxication. The blood pressure is characteristically low and the hypotension may be the first feature to bring the diagnosis under suspicion. The systemic venous pressure is raised usually with a small amplitude pulsation but occasionally tricuspid regurgitation occurs. The cardiac impulse is quiet and typically there are neither murmurs nor added sounds. In patients with a very high systemic venous pressure a right ventricular third sound is occasionally heard but tends to disappear after diuretics and a left ventricular third sound is usually conspicuously absent despite the evidence of the left ventricular failure seen on the chest x-ray.[6] Occasionally there is a murmur of mitral regurgitation.

INVESTIGATIONS

The electrocardiogram characteristically shows very low voltage particularly in the standard leads (*Figure 1*). Arrhythmias and conduction defects are common and there are usually repolarization abnormalities with T-wave inversion in the left ventricular leads. Although the ECG findings are in no way diagnostic, the low voltage in the limb leads is a consistent finding and usually sufficiently striking to suggest the diagnosis or, conversely, to make it unlikely.[6–8]

Radiography

The chest radiograph is typical if it shows little or no cardiac enlargement with marked changes of pulmonary venous congestion. This evidence of left ventricular failure makes a diagnosis of constrictive pericarditis unlikely.[6] The superior vena cava and azygos veins may be prominent, reflecting the high systemic venous pressure. Sometimes a pericardial effusion enlarges the heart shadow, obscuring the fact that the heart is quite small; the echo pictures then reveal the true position.

Echocardiography

The echocardiographic features are characteristic and reflect the functional impairment (*Figure 2*). The M-mode echo usually strongly suggests the diagnosis but 2-D echocardiograms may be virtually diagnostic because the amyloid tends to reflect the echoes giving rise to a diffuse glittering granularity of the myocardium which may be particularly dense in the endocardium. Both M-mode and 2-D show that the left ventricular cavity is of normal or reduced dimensions with

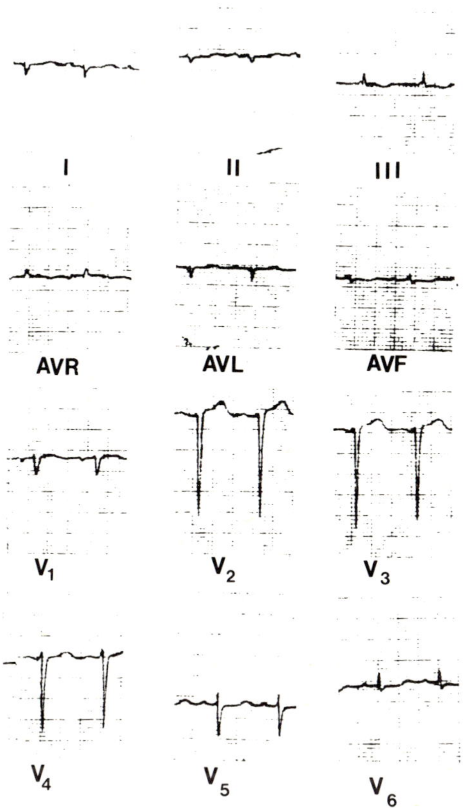

Figure 1. Typical electrocardiogram in amyloid heart disease. It shows sinus rhythm with abnormal QRS axis and extremely low voltage in the standard and limb leads.

generally diminished amplitude of excursion. Increased thickness of the right ventricle may be recognized anteriorly and a pericardial effusion may be seen in cases in which a large radiological shadow has obscured a near normal sized though abnormally contracting heart. The left ventricular wall thickness is increased symmetrically and the diminished movement is responsible also for reduced systolic thickening. Mitral valve movement is usually normal but aortic valve movement may reflect the low cardiac output, showing shortened ejection time with a tendency for the valve not to remain fully open during systole.[9, 10]

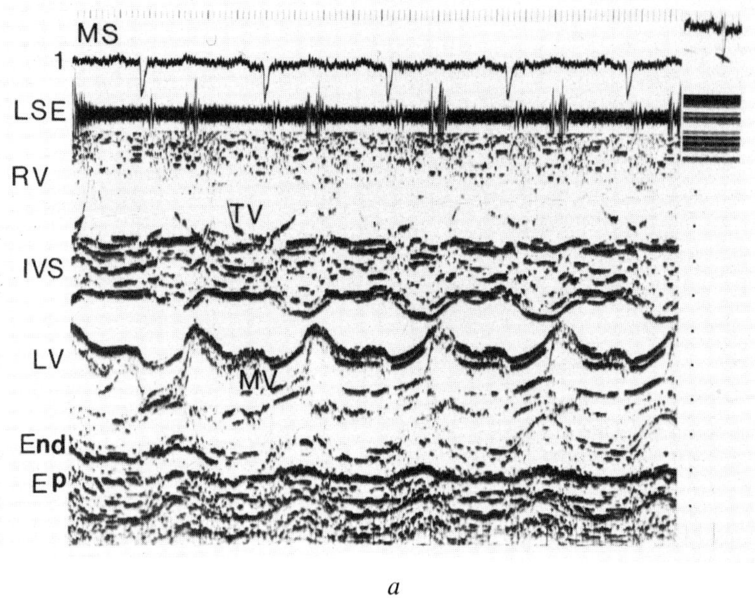

a

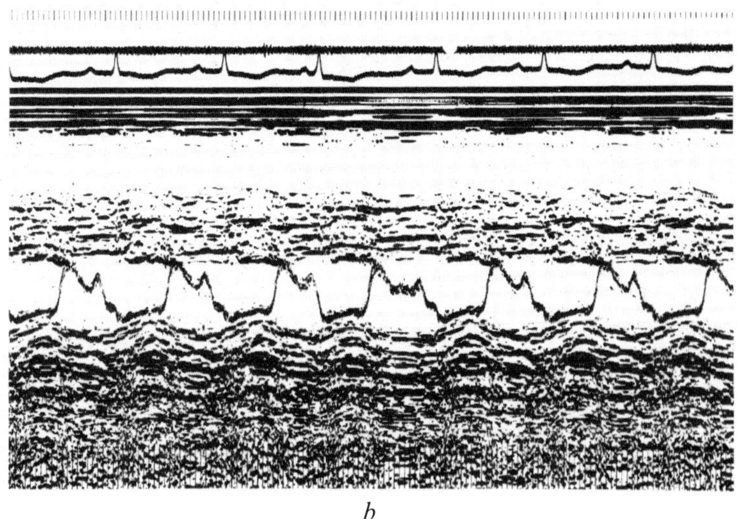

b

Figure 2. M-mode echocardiograms show small right and left ventricular cavities with very thick anterior right ventricular wall (RV) and septum (IVS). (a) The phonocardiogram (LSE) shows a widely split second sound without respiratory movement. (b) The mitral valve appears to fill the left ventricle which again has very thick walls (vertical 1 cm scale is seen to right of (a)).

Haemodynamic Tests

The haemodynamic abnormalities are also characteristic. The stroke volume is exceedingly low. There is sometimes moderate pulmonary hypertension. The diastolic pressures are high in both ventricles but the pressure is usually very much higher in the left ventricle than in the right ventricle (*Figure 3a*). Although the diastolic contour may suggest a dip and plateau form the diastolic pressure differs from that in constrictive pericarditis because the beginning pressure is also high and after an early rapid rise in pressure there is a continued slow rise rather than a plateau and there may also be a prominent a-wave (*Figure 3b*).[6,11]

Angiography

Left and right ventricular angiography may superficially look rather normal (*Figure 4a*) but the left ventricle characteristically shows rather a shaggy outline with coarsened trabeculations and exaggerated papillary muscle indentations caused by the amyloid infiltration (*Figure 4b*), and the ejection fraction is usually at the lower limit of normal or below it with a normal or small end-diastolic volume, the reduced difference between them being responsible for the very low stroke volume. Mitral regurgitation is occasionally seen.[6,12]

Biopsy

The diagnosis of cardiac amyloid can be confirmed by endomyocardial biopsy (*Figure 5*).[13]

TREATMENT

So far there is no way known to halt the progression of the amyloid infiltration. Colchicine which is effective in familial Mediterranean fever does not work in primary amyloidosis, and cytotoxic drugs given for myeloma have not been shown to have any influence on the progression of the associated amyloid heart disease. There has been a recent suggestion that large doses of vitamin C may help to activate an 'amyloid degrading factor' present in normal serum but reduced or absent in patients with amyloidosis; supportive clinical evidence is lacking. The prognosis is very poor, usually less than a year after the onset of heart failure.[14]

DIFFERENTIAL DIAGNOSIS

Differential diagnosis of the heart disease is from coronary heart disease, other forms of heart muscle disease and from constrictive pericarditis.[15–23]

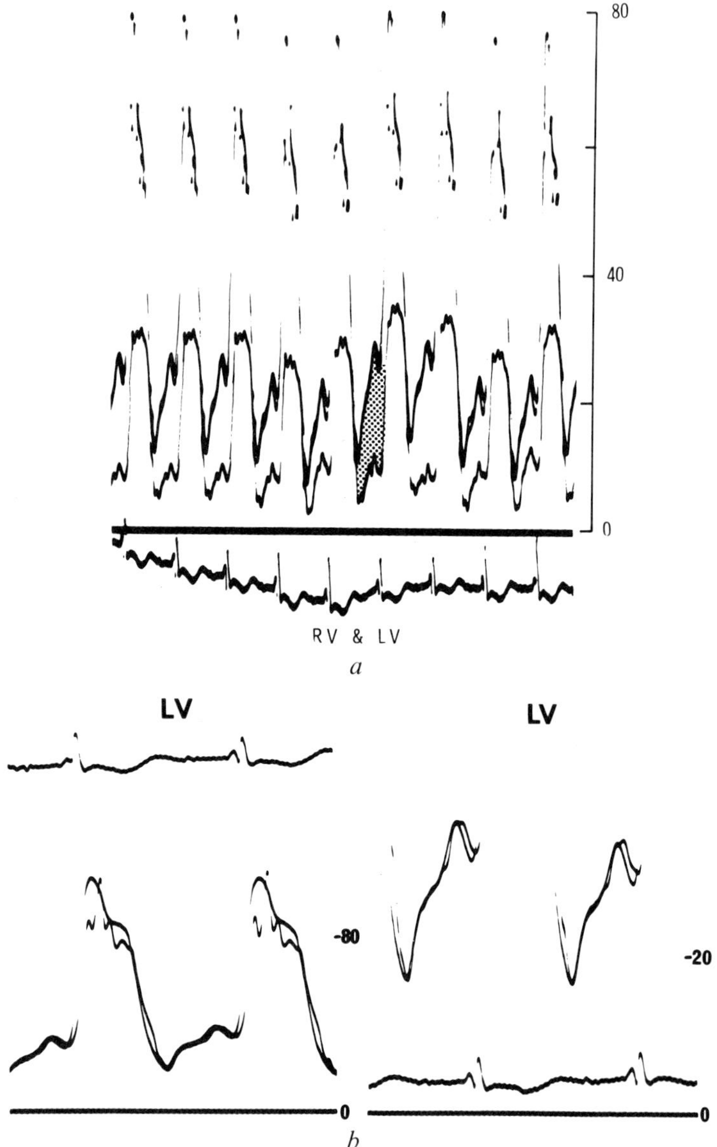

Figure 3. Simultaneously recorded left (LV) and right (RV) ventricular pressure traces showing low systolic LV pressure and raised RV pressure with diastolic pressures raised throughout diastole and considerably more in the LV than in the RV. In (b) the LV pressure is seen with the characteristic shape of the diastolic LV pressure shown in the right hand trace. (Pressures in (b) were recorded with manometer tipped catheter and the high fidelity trace is seen superimposed on that through the fluid filled catheter. Scale in mm Hg shown on the right.)

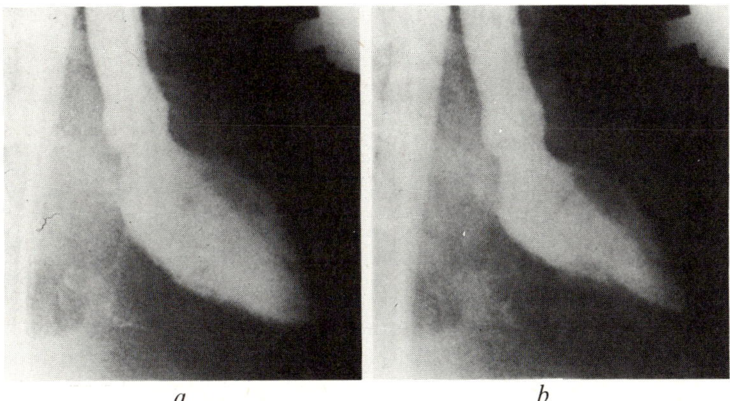

Figure 4. Left ventricular angiograms in right anterior oblique views. (a) Shows a rather poorly contracting LV of normal shape and with no mitral reflux. (b) Shows a left ventricle of characteristically shaggy outline, very poorly contracting and with slight mitral reflux (both end systolic frames).

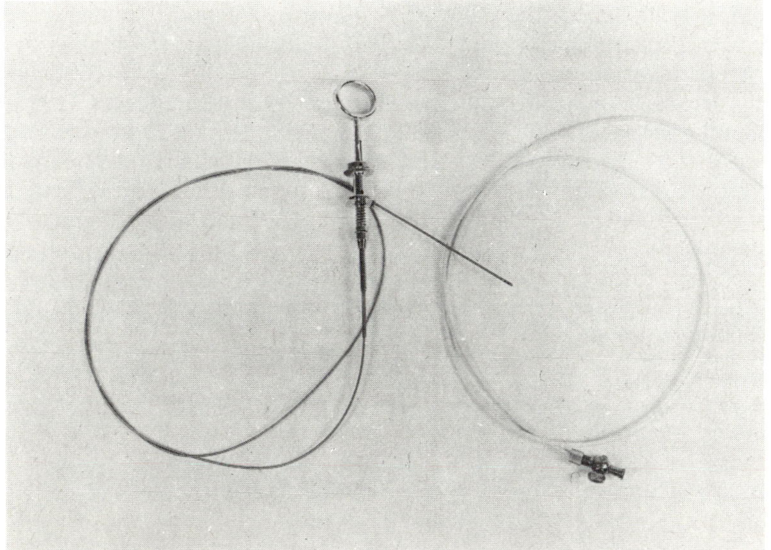

Figure 5. Simple equipment for endomyocardial biopsy: an unmodified bronchoscopic bioptone which is passed to the right (or left) ventricle through a catheter sheath. The sheath itself is introduced by the Seldinger technique mounted on a cardiac catheter to provide torque and manoeuvrability.

Angina is not uncommon in cardiac amyloid but intense heart failure with a small heart and the usual lack of diagnostic focal features on the low voltage electrocardiogram, together with the absence of history of previous infarction, are differentiating features. Since the patients are usually elderly they may sometimes have accompanying coronary disease or even have had previous infarction from this cause.

Angina occurs in most of the other forms of heart muscle disease, particularly hypertrophic cardiomyopathy (HOCM) which in its non-obstructive form complicates conjestive failure and may be the chief differential diagnosis from amyloid heart disease. In both conditions the heart is thick walled but not dilated, the output low and failure present, and the angiographic appearances may be very similar. However, the ECG is usually of high voltage in hypertrophic cardiomyopathy and 2-D echo may show the amyloid sparkle. Unfortunately fibrous tissue in HOCM may also sparkle but this is usually in the septum. Biopsy differentiates with certainty.

The haemodynamic abnormality in amyloid has been likened to that in constrictive pericarditis[16,18,19,23] although in reality they are very different and the clinical distinction should be made quite easily. Similarities are congestive failure with a small heart and low ECG voltage. There the likeness ends. In amyloidosis there is usually no third heart sound whereas in constrictive pericarditis it is usually prominent and early. In constrictive pericarditis murmurs are uncommon whereas a mitral regurgitant murmur is not rare in amyloid. In amyloidosis there is invariably pulmonary congestion on the chest x-ray whereas this is absent in constrictive pericarditis. In amyloid the ECG frequently shows conduction defects and these are rare in constrictive pericarditis. In amyloid the left and right ventricular pressures are typically dissimilar, with a much higher left ventricular and left atrial pressure than occur in constrictive pericarditis, and with a high early diastolic pressure in the ventricles compared with the normal beginning diastolic pressure in constrictive pericarditis.[6,11] Finally, pulmonary hypertension does not occur in constrictive pericarditis but is not uncommon in amyloid.

REFERENCES

1. Batsakis JG. Degenerative lesions of the heart. In: Gould SE, ed. *Pathology of the heart*, 3rd ed. Springfield, Illinois: Charles C. Thomas, 1968: 484–7.
2. Buja LM, Khoi NB, Roberts WC. Clinically significant cardiac amyloidosis. Clinicophysiological findings in 15 patients. *Am J Cardiol* 1970; 26: 394.
3. Wessler S, Freedberg AS. Cardiac amyloidosis. Electrocardiographic and pathologic observations. *Arch Intern Med* 1948; **82**: 63.
4. Cassidy JT. Cardiac amyloidosis. 2 cases with digitalis sensitivity. *Ann Intern Med* 1961; **55**: 989.
5. James TN. Pathology of the cardiac conduction system in amyloidosis. *Ann Intern Med* 1965; **65**: 28.

6. Chew C, Ziady GM, Raphael MJ, Oakley CM. The functional defect in amyloid heart disease. *Am J Cardiol* 1975; **36**: 438–44.
7. Brigden W. Cardiac amyloidosis. *Progr Cardiovasc Dis* 1957; **7**: 142.
8. Josselson AH, Pruitt RD. Electrocardiographic findings in cardiac amyloidosis. *Circulation* 1953; **7**: 200.
9. Borer JS, Henry WL, Epstein SE. Echocardiographic observations in patients with systemic infiltrative disease involving the heart. *Am J Cardiol* 1977; **39**: 184–8.
10. Child JS, Levisman JA, Abbasi AS, MacAlpin RN. Echocardiographic manifestation of infiltrative cardiomyopathy. A report of seven cases due to amyloid. *Chest* 1976; **70**: 726–31.
11. Tyberg TI, Goldyer AVN, Hurst III VW, Alexander J, Largou RA. Left ventricular filling in differentiating restrictive amyloid cardiomyopathy and constrictive pericarditis. *Am J Cardiol* 1981; **47**: 791–6.
12. Kasser IS, Kennedy JW. Measurement of left ventricular volumes in man by single plane cine angiography. *Invest Radiol* 1969; **4**: 83.
13. Brooksby IAB, Swanton RH, Jenkins BS, Webb-Peploe MM. Long sheath technique for introduction of catheter tip manometer or endomyocardial bioptone into left or right heart. *Br Heart J* 1974; **36**: 908.
14. Brandt K, Cathcart ES, Cohen AS. A clinical analysis of the course and prognosis of 42 patients with amyloidosis. *Am J Med* 1969; **44**: 955.
15. Farokh A, Walsh TJ, Massie E. Amyloid heart disease. *Am J Cardiol* 1964; **13**: 750.
16. Findley JW, Adams W. Primary systemic amyloidosis simulating constrictive pericarditis. *Arch Intern Med* 1948; **81**: 342.
17. Goodwin JF. Cardiac function in primary myocardial disease. *Br Med J* 1964; **1**: 1526.
18. Gunner RM, Dillon RF, Wallyn R, Elisberg E. Physiologic and clinical similarity between primary amyloid of the heart and constrictive pericarditis. *Circulation* 1955; **12**: 827.
19. Hetzel P, Wood EH, Burchell HB. Pressure pulses in the right side of the heart in a case of amyloid disease and in a case of idiopathic heart failure simulating constrictive pericarditis. *Proc Mayo Clinic* 1953; **28**: 107.
20. Kilpatrick TR, Horack HM, Moore CB. 'Stiff Heart' Syndrome. An uncommon cause of heart failure. *Med Clin North Am* 1967; **51**: 959.
21. Kitterage RD, Finby N. Amyloid heart disease. *AJR* 1965; **95**: 662.
22. Louis P, Michiels R, Petit A, Genin R, Bastien H. Manifestations cardiaques de l'amylose. *Coeur Med Interne* 1972; **11**: 483.
23. Shabetai R, Fowler N, Guntheroth WG. The haemodynamics of cardiac tamponade and constrictive pericarditis. *Am J Cardiol* 1970; **26**: 480.

Chapter 3

Eosinophilic heart disease

Michael M. Webb-Peploe

INTRODUCTION

Although a possible association between eosinophilia, endomyocardial disease and adherent thrombi had been suggested in the late 1800s, it was not until 1936 that Löffler[1] described in detail chronic heart failure due to endomyocardial fibrosis in association with marked eosinophilia in two Swiss patients. Since then the association between eosinophilia and endomyocardial disease has come to be well recognized and has acquired a bewildering variety of names: Löffler's endocarditis parietales fibroplastica, eosinophilic leukaemia,[2] disseminated eosinophilic collagen disease,[3] endomyocardial fibrosis and eosinophilia,[4] hypereosinophilic syndrome,[5,6] fibroma of the right ventricle,[7] Löffler's eosinophilic endocarditis[8,9] and endomyocardiopathy with eosinophilia[10] (*Figure 1*).

The first report of tropical endomyocardial fibrosis (EMF) was made by Bedford and Konstam,[11] who described heart failure of unknown aetiology in West African soldiers serving in the Middle East during World War II. The hearts of these patients who came to autopsy showed 'extensive subendocardial fibrosis . . . without appreciable inflammation'. Most of the early work clarifying this entity came from Davies and his co-workers in East Africa,[12] who (*a*) adopted the descriptive term 'endomyocardial fibrosis'; (*b*) defined specific sites of mural endocardial involvement that occurred alone or in combination, and with experience could be diagnosed ante mortem; (*c*) noted that, clinically, there was mitral and/or tricuspid regurgitation that correlated with the left- and right-sided lesions found at autopsy; (*d*) pointed out that subendocardial muscle damage appeared to precede the formation of mural thrombus which then underwent organization and

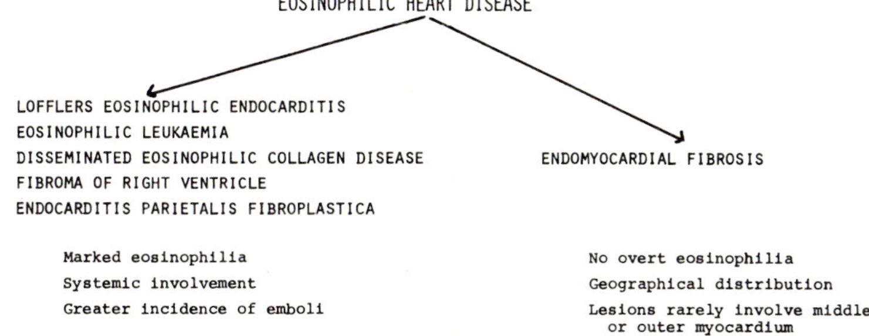

Figure 1. The distinction between Löffler's endomyocardial disease and tropical endomyocardial fibrosis is probably historical. The differences shown are probably due to earlier recognition of the condition in countries with well developed medical services. Pathologically, the two conditions are indistinguishable (see text).

fibrosis; and (*e*) observed that there was myocardial damage which was most extensive beneath the endocardial scars. The condition is not confined to Africa but has also been reported from India, Ceylon, Malaya, the Philippines, Brazil, Venezuela and Colombia. It also occurs in Europeans who have resided in the hot and humid parts of Central Africa.[13]

Controversy exists as to whether Löffler's endomyocardial disease and EMF are or are not the same condition occurring in temperate and tropical climates respectively. The many similarities—clinical, haemodynamic, angiographic and pathological—between the two conditions[9, 14] have led to the unitarian hypothesis that 'the presence of an eosinophil leucocytosis, in a susceptible person, by some unknown mechanism, causes endomyocardial damage'.[13] This concept is not uniformly accepted on the grounds that: (*a*) there is absence of eosinophilia and arteritis elsewhere in the body in EMF as there often is in Löffler's endomyocardial disease; and (*b*) the sex incidence of the two conditions is different, with females preponderating in EMF, and males in Löffler's disease. Recent careful 'blind' comparison of hearts from cases with Löffler's disease and EMF have shown no pathological differences,[15] however, supporting the unitarian hypothesis that these two conditions have the same aetiology.

AETIOLOGY

Any hypothesis has to reconcile the following observations:

1. Myocardial damage has been reported in certain diseases other than Löffler's heart disease which are characterized by increased eosinophil counts (e.g. filariasis, trichinosis and the early stages of some acute leukaemias).

2. Patients with long standing eosinophilia may, however, have no evidence of cardiac dysfunction.
3. A form of cardiomyopathy similar to that seen in Löffler's disease and EMF has been described in patients without increased eosinophil counts.[16]
4. Eosinophilia has been reported in about 30 per cent of cases of EMF in many series.
5. Tropical eosinophilia, producing pulmonary symptoms and infiltrates (common in India, Pakistan and Ceylon and due almost certainly to a non-human filarial infestation), rarely causes cardiac damage.[17]

One such hypothesis is that the cardiac damage is not dependent on the numbers of circulating eosinophils, but on whether they are normal or abnormal. Morphological abnormalities (vacuoles, reduced numbers of specific granules in the cytoplasm) are common in the circulating eosinophils of patients with endomyocardial disease.[10,18] Among the potentially cardiotoxic agents which such abnormal eosinophils might be releasing are their cationic proteins, and persistently high serum levels of eosinophilic cationic protein have been found in patients with Löffler's endomyocardial disease.[15] In addition, a number of immunological abnormalities have been described in both EMF,[19] and Löffler's disease,[20] some of which may play a role in the myocardial damage.

PATHOLOGY[21]

Three major histopathological patterns of disease may be recognized depending on the length of time between onset of disease and death of the patient:

1. Necrotic—interval between onset of symptoms and death measured in weeks. An eosinophilic myocarditis with particular involvement of the inner layers of the myocardium and arteritis of small intramural vessels is characteristic. Areas of myocardial necrosis are present.
2. Thrombotic—interval between onset of symptoms and death measured in months. Thrombus is frequently present and there is prominent fibrous endocardial thickening which may be continuous with myocardial scars (presumably the fibrosed necrotic areas noted in the necrotic stage). Arteritis still persists.
3. Fibrotic—interval between onset of symptoms and death measured in years. Thick fibrous endocardium with some superimposed thrombus is characteristic, and the thickened endocardium shows zonal layering: superficial layer of hyaline collagen, middle layer of fibrous tissue, and deepest layer showing varying degrees of chronic inflammatory cell infiltration with varying numbers of eosinophils and dilated blood vessels.

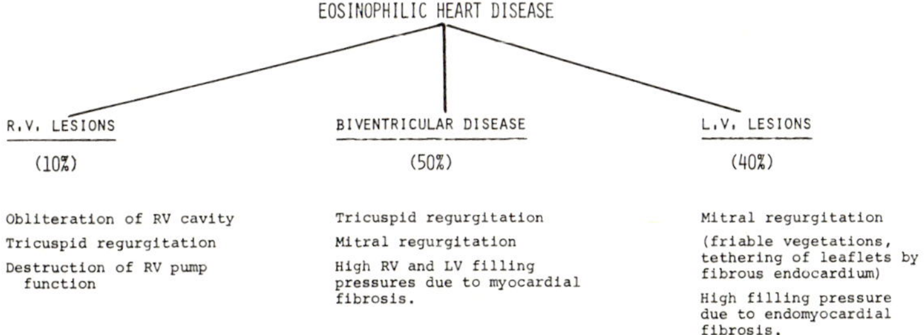

Figure 2. Cardiovascular findings in eosinophilic heart disease.

CARDIOVASCULAR FINDINGS[6,9,22] (*Figure 2*)

The symptoms and signs depend on whether the disease process affects principally the right ventricle (approximately 10 per cent), both ventricles (approximately 50 per cent) or the left ventricle (about 40 per cent). In right ventricular disease, hepatomegaly, ascites and peripheral oedema, together with elevation of the central venous pressure and signs of tricuspid regurgitation, are characteristic. In biventricular disease, in addition to the right ventricular signs, there is pulmonary venous congestion causing cough, progressive dyspnoea of effort and sometimes haemoptysis, together with evidence of pulmonary arterial hypertension and mitral regurgitation. Patients with predominantly left ventricular involvement present with signs of mitral regurgitation and pulmonary hypertension, and characteristically it is the posterior mitral chordae and papillary muscle that are involved by the endomyocardial fibrotic process, the anterior sub-valve apparatus still having a normal function.

INVESTIGATIONS

The Electrocardiogram

The ECG can be normal (up to 35 per cent of cases), but characteristically shows low voltage QRS, non-specific T wave changes, a P mitrale and right axis deviation.

Chest Radiograph

The heart size is often normal or only slightly enlarged (unless there is predominant right ventricular involvement with marked right atrial dilatation), and there may be evidence of pulmonary venous congestion with, in some cases, pleural effusions. In EMF affecting the right ventricle there may be calcification of the fibrosed right ventricular apex.

Echocardiography

In patients with the hypereosinophilic syndrome symmetrical thickening of the left ventricular wall, without an increase in diastolic cavity dimension in a normotensive patient with signs of left ventricular failure were characteristic and strongly suggestive of a restrictive cardiomyopathy process involving the left ventricle. Ejection fraction was well preserved.[6] In those cases with right ventricular involvement there is paradoxical septal motion, implying (in the presence of right heart failure) right ventricular volume overload. Usually in such circumstances the tricuspid valve and right ventricular cavity are well seen, but in endomyocardial disease the extensive obliteration of the right ventricular cavity and tethering of the tricuspid valve leaflets prevents their identification.[9]

Haemodynamics

The haemodynamic and angiographic features of Löffler's endomyocardial disease[4,7–10] and EMF[23,24] are identical. In those cases with left ventricular or biventricular disease, left atrial or pulmonary wedge pressures are raised due to a combination of mitral regurgitation and restriction of left ventricular filling by endomyocardial fibrosis. There is often severe pulmonary hypertension. Left ventricular angiography confirms the mitral regurgitation (often through the posterior part of the valve) and may show mural thrombus particularly of the apex. Abnormalities of the large coronary arteries are occasionally seen on coronary arteriography, but are probably due to coincidental atheromatous disease rather than forming an integral part of the endomyocardial disease process. The cardiac output is well maintained until a late stage of the disease.

In those cases with right ventricular involvement alone, left heart pressures may be normal, but right ventricular contraction produces no measurable effect on the right-sided pressures due to extensive right ventricular cavity obliteration. This results in very similar pressures being recorded from pulmonary artery, right ventricle and right atrium (*Figure 3*). Right ventricular angiograms confirm the obliteration of the ventricular cavity and the presence of severe tricuspid regurgitation (*Figure 4*).

Endomyocardial Biopsy

It is often difficult to obtain specimens as the bioptome slides over the smooth fibrous endocardium but, when successful, organized thrombus or fibrosis are characteristic.[9,25]

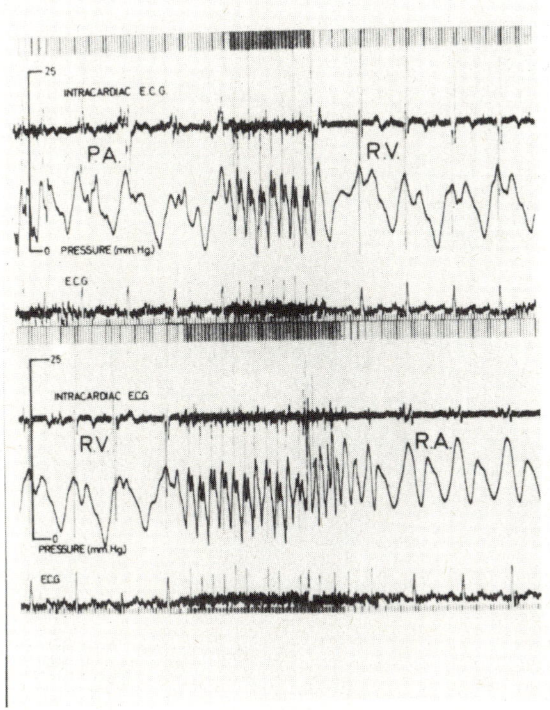

Figure 3. Pressure withdrawal from pulmonary artery (PA) to right ventricle (RV)—upper panel, and from right ventricle (RV) to right atrium (RA)—lower panel, in a case of Löffler's endomyocardial disease. Note that although the intracardiac ECG (top tracing) shows the expected changes on passing from PA to RV to RA, the pressures in these three sites (middle tracings) are virtually identical.

NATURAL HISTORY

Patients typically describe the insidious onset of increasingly severe symptoms of left or right heart failure. Sudden death, syncopal episodes and arrhythmias are uncommon. Although mural thrombus formation is a common pathological finding, overt systemic or pulmonary embolism is relatively uncommon. However, because there is often autopsy evidence of emboli to many different organs, all patients with endomyocardial disease should be considered for long-term anticoagulant therapy. In most reports, patients with this condition respond

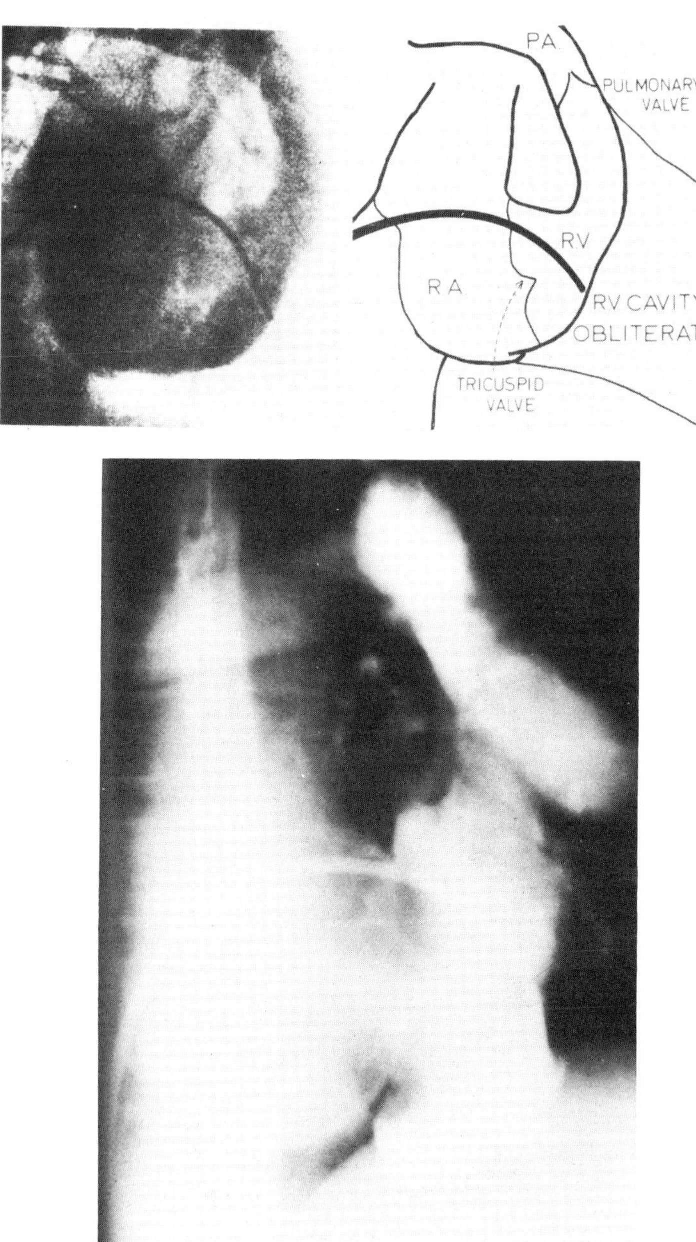

Figure 4. Right ventricular ciné-angiograms in two cases of Löffler's endomyocardial disease both showing extensive obliteration of the cavity of the right ventricle.

poorly to treatment and the process of progressive endomyocardial fibrosis ends fatally in several months to several years. Bacterial endocarditis is a very unusual complication.

TREATMENT

Medical

Treatment with digitalis and diuretics alone is usually only of temporary benefit in the face of the inexorable advance of the endomyocardial fibrosis. Anti-hypereosinophilic therapy with hydroxyurea and/or steroids has been found to arrest or reverse the clinical and echocardiographic manifestations of some cases of Löffler's endomyocardial disease.[6,26] In other reports[9,10] such treatment has been disappointing, although it can be argued that the therapy in these cases was not sufficiently intensive, since there was little or no reduction in eosinophil count.

Surgical

Reports of surgical treatment of both Löffler's endomyocardial disease[9,27] and tropical endomyocardial fibrosis[28–32] are beginning to appear in the literature. Such surgery involves repair or replacement of the mitral valve, repair of the tricuspid valve or its replacement, and decortication in those cases of extensive obliteration of the ventricular cavities. The few patients who have undergone successful surgery appear to improve symptomatically, but follow-up is too short and the numbers too small to permit assessment of the effect of surgery on life expectancy.

REFERENCES

1. Löffler W. Endocarditis parietalis fibroplastica mit Bluteosinophilie. *Schweiz Med Wochenschr* 1936; **17**: 817.
2. Bentley HP, Reardon AE, Knoedler JP, Krivit W. Eosinophilic leukaemia. *Am J Med* 1961; **30**: 310.
3. Engfeldt B, Zetterström R. Disseminated eosinophilic 'collagen disease'. *Acta Med Scand* 1956; **153**: 337.
4. Roberts WC, Liegler DG, Carbone PP. Endomyocardial disease and eosinophilia: a clinical and pathological spectrum. *Am J Med* 1969; **46**: 28.
5. Hardy WR, Anderson RE. The hypereosinophilic syndromes. *Ann Intern Med* 1968; **68**: 1220.
6. Parillo JE, Borer JS, Henry WL, Wolff SM, Fauci AS. The cardiovascular manifestations of the hypereosinophilic syndrome. *Am J Med* 1979; **67**: 572.
7. Van der Hauwaert LG, Corbed L, Maldague P. Fibroma of the right ventricle producing severe tricuspid stenosis. *Circulation* 1968; **32**: 451.
8. Gardner-Thorpe G, Harriman DGF, Parsons M, Rudge P. Löffler's eosinophilic endocarditis with Balint's syndrome (optic ataxia and paralysis of visual fixation). *Q J Med* 1971; **40**: 249.

9. Bell JA, Jenkins BS, Webb-Peploe MM. Clinical, haemodynamic and angiographic findings in Löffler's eosinophilic endocarditis. *Br Heart J* 1976; **38**: 541.
10. Solley GO, Maldonado JE, Gleich GJ et al. Endomyocardiopathy with eosinophilia. *Mayo Clin Proc* 1976; **51**: 697.
11. Bedford DE, Konstam GLS. Heart failure of unknown aetiology in Africans. *Br Heart J* 1946; **8**: 236.
12. Ball JD, Williams AW, Davies JNP. Endomyocardial fibrosis. *Lancet* 1954; **1**: 1049.
13. Brockington ID, Olsen EGJ, Goodwin JF. Endomyocardial fibrosis in Europeans resident in tropical Africa. *Lancet* 1959; **1**: 583.
14. Anonymous. Sinister eosinophils in the heart? *Lancet* 1977; **1**: 943.
15. Olsen EGJ, Spry CJS. The pathogenesis of Löffler's endomyocardial disease and its relationship to endomyocardial fibrosis. In: Yu PN, Goodwin JF, eds. *Progress in cardiology*, vol. 8. Philadelphia: Lea & Febiger, 1979: 281.
16. Roberts WC, Ferrans VJ. Pathological aspects of certain cardiomyopathies. *Circ Res* 1974; **34**: **35**: (Suppl. II) II-128.
17. Johny KV, Ananthachari MD. Cardiovascular changes in tropical eosinophilia. *Am Heart J* 1965; **69**: 59.
18. Spry CJF, Tai PC. Studies on blood eosinophils II. Patients with Löffler's cardiomyopathy. *Clin Exp Immunol* 1976; **24**: 423.
19. Shaper AG, Kaplan MH, Foster WD et al. Immunological studies in endomyocardial fibrosis and other forms of heart disease in the tropics. *Lancet* 1967; **1**: 598.
20. Parillo JE, Lawley T, Frank MM et al. Immune reactivity in the hypereosinophilic syndrome. *J Allergy Clin Immunol* 1979; **64**: 113.
21. Olsen EGJ. Endomyocardial fibrosis and Löffler's endocarditis parietalis fibroplastica. *Postgrad Med. J* 1977; **53**: 538.
22. Connor DH, Somers K, Hutt MSR et al. Endomyocardial fibrosis in Uganda: an epidemiological, clinical and pathologic study. *Am Heart J* 1967; Pt. I: **74**: 687. 1968; Pt. II: **75**: 107.
23. Fowler JM, Somers K. Left ventricular endomyocardial fibrosis and mitral incompetence. *Lancet* 1968; **1**: 227.
24. Somers K, Brenton DP, D'Arbela PG et al. Haemodynamic features of severe endomyocardial fibrosis of the right ventricle including comparison with constrictive pericarditis. *Br Heart J* 1968; **30**: 322.
25. Somers K, Hutt MSR, Patel AK, D'Arbela PG. Endomyocardial biopsy in diagnosis of cardiomyopathies. *Br Heart J* 1971; **33**: 822.
26. Parrillo JE, Fauci AS, Wolff SM. Therapy of the hypereosinophilic syndrome. *Ann Intern Med* 1978; **89**: 167.
27. Weyman AE, Rankin R, King M. Löffler's endocarditis presenting as mitral and tricuspid stenoses. *Am J Cardiol* 1977; **40**: 438.
28. Hess OM, Turina M, Senning A et al. Pre- and post-operative findings in patients with endomyocardial fibrosis. *Br Heart J* 1978; **40**: 406.
29. Lepley O Jr., Avis A, Korns ME et al. Endomyocardial fibrosis. A surgical approach. *Ann Thorac Surg* 1974; **18**: 626.
30. Dubost C, Maurice P, Gerbaux A et al. The surgical treatment of constrictive fibrous endocarditis. *Ann Surg* 1976; **184**: 303.
31. Dubost C, Maurice P, Gerbaux A et al. L'endocardite fibreuse constrictive. Traitement chirurgical. *Arch Mal Coeur* 1977; **70**: 155.
32. Sheikhzadeh AH, Tarbiat S, Nazarian T et al. Constrictive endocarditis. Report of a case with successful surgery. *Br Heart J* 1979; **42**: 224.

Chapter 4

Cardiac disease associated with iron overload

Andrew G. Mitchell

The heart disease seen in haemochromatosis is rare but of considerable interest since there is evidence that it is one of the few reversible causes of myocardial cell damage. The accumulation of iron as a pathological process culminates in the clinical picture of haemochromatosis. This may be defined as a chronic disease state in which there are excessive deposits of iron in a variety of organs leading to functional impairment.[1] When no functional impairment occurs, the term haemosiderosis is more appropriate.

A number of underlying processes may lead to the iron accumulation, and it is conventional to consider separately primary, or idiopathic, haemochromatosis and the secondary forms. However, the damaging effects of iron appear similar in both groups. With rare diseases it is not easy to maintain uniformity within the population studied, and this remains true for haemochromatosis. With the idiopathic form, the aetiology appears to be a genetically determined increase of iron absorption by the intestines. There is an association with HLA groups A3 and B14 and abnormalities of iron absorption may be noted in a proportion of close relatives.[2] The serum ferritin may be a useful indicator of this genetic marker.[3] Apart from a wide age distribution, from 20 years upwards, with its attendant degenerative processes, this group is homogenous. The most frequent form of secondary haemochromatosis occurs as a result of chronic blood transfusions for non-haemorrhagic anaemias. This forms a much less uniform group, with a wide scatter of ages, and degrees and types of anaemia. Within this group are more homogenous populations and part of this Chapter will relate to the follow-up of a group of children with beta-thalassaemia observed at the Royal Free Hospital over a period of many years. Although some cases of iron overload may be associated with alcoholism, there is no evidence that the cardiac disease seen in haemochromatosis is dependent upon the alcohol intake.

Sufficient accumulation of iron to cause haemochromatosis is a relatively rare occurrence. Estimates of the incidence of idiopathic haemochromatosis range from 4 to 25 per 100 000 necropsies.[1] In this situation the iron is derived totally from dietary sources and, assuming complete uptake of ingested iron, would take at least 15–20 years to develop. It is largely a disease of males. The frequency of secondary haemochromatosis is very difficult to assess. When associated with anaemia the iron accumulation is largely due to the iron content of transfused blood, although increased absorption of dietary iron may also play a part when there is marked marrow hyperplasia.[4] The iron load of 1 unit of blood is approximately 250 mg, and important cardiac damage requires generally in excess of 100 units transfused.

There is now extensive information about normal iron metabolism.[1] For this Chapter, it is sufficient to mention a few details concerning the methods of removing iron from the body stores. Iron, which is transported in the body as transferrin, has an ability to exchange with the iron stored as ferritin and the more insoluble polymer haemosiderin. The transferrin is used by the marrow to form haemoglobin. Chelating agents, such as desferrioxamine mesylate, are able to remove iron from the circulation and possibly from an intracellular pool with excretion in the bile and urine. The degree of chelation may be increased by the administration of ascorbic acid. Prolonged infusions of desferrioxamine are generally more effective than similar doses given as a bolus, and the regimes used may differ substantially. Our regime for thalassaemic children is to infuse 200 mg subcutaneously overnight, with oral supplements of ascorbic acid. Other regimes have used intramuscular injections of the chelating agent.

There is no doubt that therapeutic measures can remove the majority of the iron load in haemochromatosis. The total iron content in haemochromatosis is 20–60 g compared with the normal 4–5 g, and removal of the iron leads to clear improvement of liver structure and function.[5,6] Measurement of the iron content of the liver from biopsy specimens gives a useful guide to the total body iron and consequently to the duration of therapy initially required. It is not sufficient to use the appearance of an iron deficient picture on the blood film as a guide to depletion of total stores.

The mechanisms by which iron causes myocardial cell damage remain unproven. However, free iron radicles, possibly released from degraded ferritin, stimulate lipid peroxidation of lysosymal and other intracellular membranes. In the liver of idiopathic haemochromatosis, lysosymes appear to be particularly fragile.[7] Ascorbic acid increases the lipid peroxidation and so, in theory, may aggravate cellular damage.

The degree to which the iron directly causes the myocardial cell impairment, as opposed to focal necrosis leading to fibrous replacement within the heart, remains unclear and yet is crucial to the likelihood of reversibility of the cardiac problem.

Patients with haemochromatosis often present with the classic triad of hepatomegaly, diabetes mellitus and skin pigmentation. The diabetes may become resistant to insulin. Additionally, evidence of other hormone deficiencies may occur, particularly gonadal and pituitary failure. Impotence and loss of libido are common and testicular atrophy can be found in about three-quarters of cases. Splenomegaly may occur in about one-quarter of cases.[1] Chondrocalcinosis should be looked for radiologically. In general the liver disease has a prolonged and relatively benign course, but systemic evidence of liver disease should not be overlooked and liver failure may develop. Malignant hepatoma may occur, particularly in the older patients. Cardiac involvement may occur in the absence of these features, including even diabetes or hepatomegaly. The diagnosis is supported by a high serum iron generally in excess of 27 micromoles per litre and with at least 75 per cent saturation of transferrin. The serum ferritin is a guide to the total body iron, and levels above 1000 mg/ml are virtually diagnostic. However, the most reliable method is liver biopsy, giving a histological picture, together with assay of the iron content which gives a good guide to the total of body iron. Severe hepatic involvement may occur with little or no clinical cardiac impairment. Cardiac biopsy will demonstrate the iron infiltration in the heart, but is generally indicated only when there is a serious cardiac problem.

Prior to the availability of insulin, the mortality of haemochromatosis was dominated by diabetic complications. However, by 1955 the importance of heart failure was recognized as a major cause of death in idiopathic haemochromatosis.[8,9] Thirty per cent of cases died in heart failure and, for the age group 30–40 years, the incidence of heart failure doubled. The life expectancy was under 2 years when the disease presented before the age of 30 years. Other more recent studies have suggested a lower incidence of heart failure as the cause of death,[5] although to some extent differences may be due to the ages of the population studied. It is uncommon for idiopathic haemochromatosis to present before the age of 40 years, although this is not true for the transfusional forms where death from cardiac failure often occurs in the second or third decade. Improvement in survival as a result of venesection has been shown, but some of these series had a low incidence of cardiac complications overall.[10–12] More encouraging from the cardiac aspect are isolated reports of the resolution of heart failure with adequate venesection therapy.[13–15]

Cardiac involvement is an important feature in 15 per cent of cases of haemochromatosis and may be detected in many more in the absence of adequate preventative therapy.[12] The clinical picture is dominated either by heart failure or more often by arrhythmias. The former usually resembles the pattern of a dilated cardiomyopathy with biventricular failure, gallop rhythms, atrio-ventricular valve incompetence and clinical and radiological cardiomegaly. The appearance of heart failure has indicated a poor outlook with few cases surviving over 1 or 2 years untreated. The history in some of the most severe cases of heart failure is often short with a rapid downhill course, giving little time for the diagnosis to be established and significant amounts of iron to be mobilized. Particularly important is the right ventricular element in a proportion of cases and ascites and oedema may be aggravated by liver impairment. Haemodynamic parameters are infrequently documented in the literature, although probably are similar to other forms of dilated cardiomyopathy.[12] Impaired ventricular function may also be demonstrated by systolic time intervals.

A proportion of cases are described as showing a 'restrict' picture.[16–18] The initial case described underwent exploration for constrictive pericarditis and during surgery the diastolic pressure trace in the right ventricle showed a 'dip and plateau' pattern. However, the diagnosis of haemochromatosis was not straightforward, for the patient was known to be an alcoholic and the serum iron was not as high as is usually seen. The haemodynamic features demonstrated by Cutler include a prominent 'Y' descent in the right atrium, a marked dip in the right ventricular diastolic pressure to zero, and approximation of the mean right atrial pressure, right ventricular and pulmonary diastolic pressures and mean wedge pressure. The low right ventricular minimum diastolic pressure resembled constriction but the later diastolic pressures continued to rise and did not show a marked plateau formation. This picture is not typical of either constriction or the restrictive picture of amyloid heart disease,[19] but this case may not be representative.

The haemodynamic findings in a recent case of severe cardiomyopathy showing some restrictive features is illustrated (*Figures 1* and *2*). Severe venous congestion was accompanied by a sharp diastolic fall of the jugular pulse. There was little cardiomegaly with a quiet ventricular impulse, and left ventricular diastolic dimensions on echocardiography remained just within normal limits. The soft gallop rhythm appeared to be right ventricular in origin. The right ventricular diastolic pressure showed a 'dip and plateau' pattern but with a minimum pressure of 12 mm Hg. There was approximation of both mean atrial pressures and the right ventricular and pulmonary artery diastolic pressure (*Figure 1*). However, clear differences from constrictive pericarditis could be demonstrated. Angiographically and echocardiographically, there was marked depression of systolic function with an ejection fraction of 35 per cent and slow but definite ventricular filling throughout diastole.

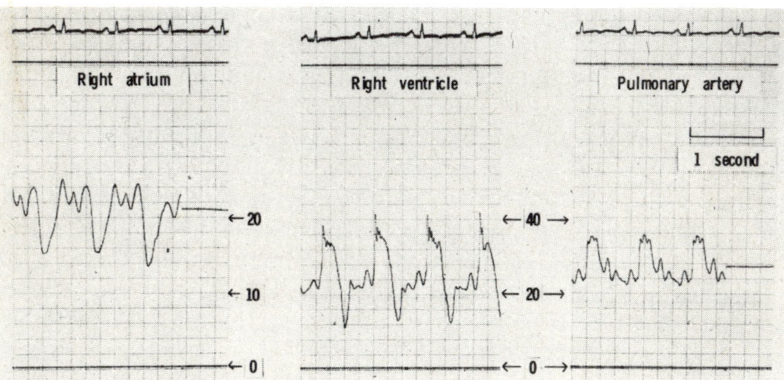

Figure 1. Right heart pressures in 'restrictive' pattern of haemochromatosis heart disease. The 'dip and plateau' pattern in the right ventricle is also seen in the atrium but the minimum diastolic pressure is high. Pressures in mm Hg.

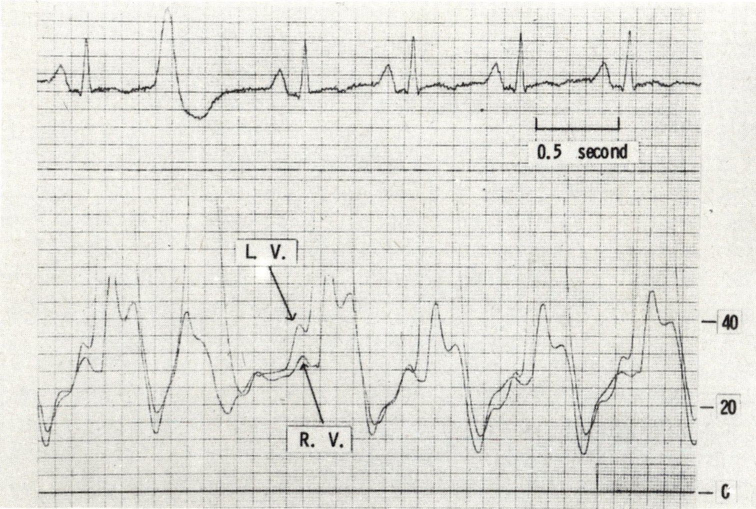

Figure 2. Simultaneous right and left ventricular pressure traces, from the same case as Fig. 1, showing the small end diastolic difference increased following a ventricular premature beat.

Although the end diastolic pressures in the ventricles did not differ by more than 6 mm Hg, the 'dip and plateau' effect was less clear in the left ventricle, and atrial contraction waves were more prominent in the left ventricular trace than the right (*Figure 2*). Changes in fluid loading as a result of radiographic contrast media or venesection had greater effects on right-sided filling than on the left ventricular response. As in other forms of restrictive cardiomyopathy, I believe careful analysis of the systolic and diastolic function will distinguish these muscle faults from external constriction.

A relationship with pericardial disease occurs in a number of other cases[12,20,21] and two cases are described, without further details, as having previously having pericardectomy.[20] Whether the acute pericarditis is a feature of iron toxicity is not clear as many of the reported cases occurred after splenectomy, which may predispose to viral infection. Angina-like pain may occur and while the coronary arteries are generally free of obstructive atheroma, this is not invariable, particularly in the older age group.[5] Angina has been noted to regress with iron depletion by venesection, although the coronary anatomy was not defined in the particular case.[22]

With regard to rhythm disturbances, supraventricular and ventricular arrhythmias are frequent and occasionally may be life-threatening. Ambulatory monitoring demonstrates arrhythmias in about half of the cases with some reduction in the frequency of premature beats when chelation therapy is well maintained (personal communication). Conduction disturbances may also occur[12,23] and all degrees of atrio-ventricular block and bundle branch block have been described. Symptomatic heart block may require permanent pacing and there is, as yet, no indication that removal of iron from the heart reverses the conduction problem. The surface ECG usually suggests the block to be in the region of the atrio-ventricular node, and available electro-physiological evidence supports this view.[12,24] However, abnormal atrio-ventricular conduction with normal surface ECG conduction has also been described, and electrical stimulation studies of cardiac conduction might be expected to show abnormalities in a high proportion of cases. The resting ECG may show a variety of repolarization changes, including elevation or depression of the ST segment, T-wave flattening or inversion and occasionally Q-T prolongation. Low voltage recordings in the frontal plane are common (*Figures 3* and *4*). These changes are in no way specific and may be seen in many forms of widespread myocardial damage and also in pericardial constriction.

The correlation between the ECG findings and the histology of the conducting system is poor.[25] Iron appears more prominently in the atrio-ventricular node than the sino-atrial node, but the density in the conduction tissues is often less than that of the surrounding muscle. However, atrio-ventricular node deposits are always dense when heart block is present. The deposition of iron is readily shown by Perl's stain (*Figure 5*); the majority of iron lies membrane-bound within the myocardial cells and there is very little interstitial iron. Initially the perinuclear region of the myocardial cell is involved but, as the iron

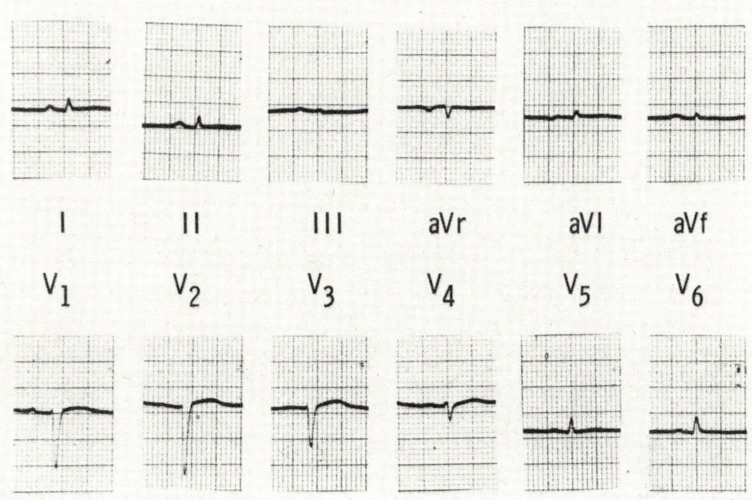

Figure 3. Low voltage QRS and T waves in haemochromatosis heart disease (male 42 years).

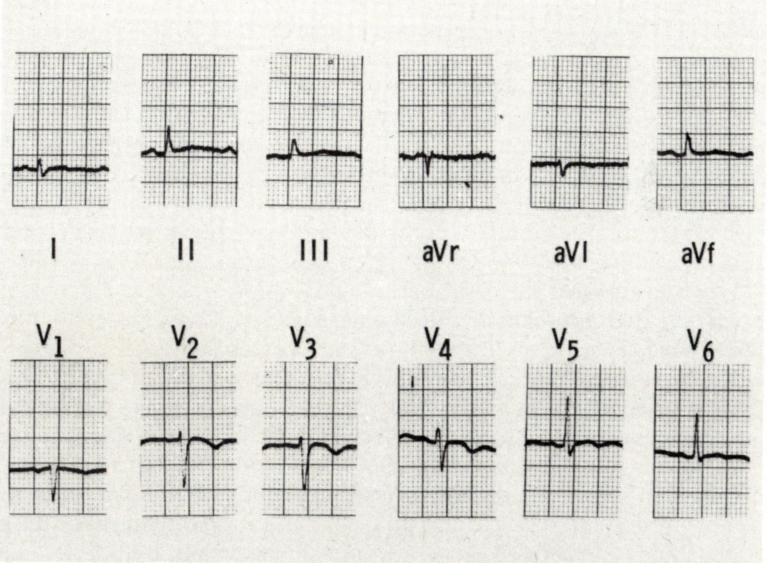

Figure 4. Widespread ST and T wave changes in haemochromatosis heart disease. The praecordial changes appeared over 2 weeks with the development of congestive heart failure. There was no evidence of ischaemic heart disease (male 54 years).

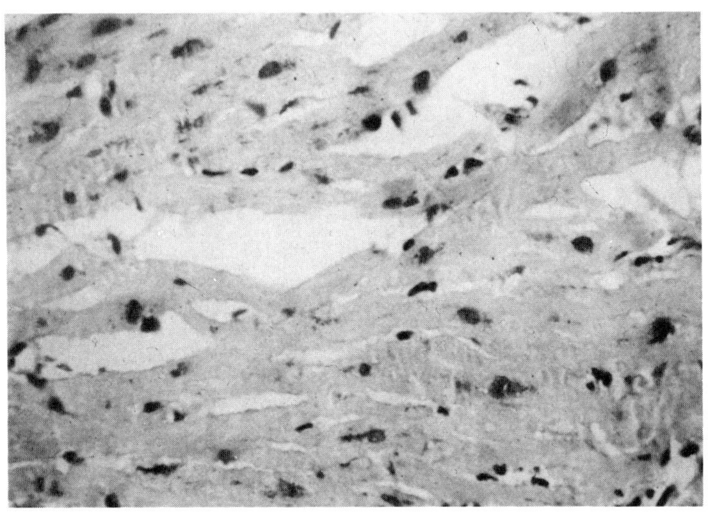

Figure 5. Perl's stain of endomyocardial biopsy in haemochromatosis heart disease showing gross iron deposition but no increase of interstitial fibrous tissue (magnification × 40).

overload increases, a greater proportion of the myocardial cell is affected. The electron microscope has shown that these deposits are related at least in part to lysosomal particles. The iron is generally widely distributed through the heart with the greatest concentration in the epicardium and more involvement in the ventricles than in the atria.[26] The iron content of the right and left ventricles at 3000–4000 μg/g of dry tissue is ten times the normal level. Iron content in the atria is about half that in the ventricles. For secondary haemochromatosis comparable figures are available in only one case and were rather less than for the idiopathic forms.[12,24]

For transfusional siderosis, pathological studies indicate differences occurring after approximately 100 units of blood. Cases exceeding this figure have extensive involvement with macroscopically visible changes in the heart unless there is, in addition, an element of blood loss.[26] This pattern of involvement of the heart is usually accompanied by clinical and ECG evidence of cardiac involvement. When the iron deposits are only detectable microscopically then heart failure and ECG changes are unusual and transient, and probably are not more frequent than in a controlled group with chronic anaemia. The approximate separation at 100 units of transfused blood may not be universally applicable. The iron content in three of four cases of secondary haemochromatosis undergoing endomyocardial biopsy was only marginally increased above normal in spite of at least 150 units of transfused blood.[27] Since the subendocardial muscle generally has the least accumulation of iron, the use of transvenous biopsy material may not always be reliable.

In severe haemochromatosis affecting the heart there is marked dilatation of all four chambers with considerable increase in the weight of the heart. The muscle appears as a rusty brown colour and ventricular hypertrophy is not prominent. Mural thrombi may occur without evidence of underlying infarction, although systemic embolism has not been reported. Fibrosis within the myocardium is variable and often mild and does not correlate closely with the functional impairment. There may be areas of myofibrillar destruction and marked variation of cell size, but relatively little necrosis of myocytes. This lack of extensive permanent damage, even when death has occurred from severe cardiac failure, has supported the theory that the iron has a more direct toxic or metabolic effect on the myocyte. This clearly must involve both the contracting and relaxing properties of the heart. There is always severe iron loading of the liver and of other organs and occasionally cirrhosis may develop. There appear to be important differences in the response of the liver to iron loading where interstitial deposition and fibrosis are more prominent than in the heart.

Haemochromatosis heart disease should not be considered simply as the static picture described above. There is a long continuing process of iron accumulation, together with interventions aimed at reversing this process. Echocardiography may be used to document changes in ventricular function over a period of time. Deterioration in an individual may be shown as an increase in ventricular diastolic diameter and a fall of ejection fraction.[24] In a number of cases of transfusional haemochromatosis, progressive dilatation of the ventricle, together with clinical deterioration, has been attributed to the addition of ascorbic acid to the chelation therapy, and this effect appears to be reversible.[28] In contrast, a fall of ventricular dimensions has been noted to accompany clinical improvement and iron removal by venesection.[13] In our own series of 17 children with thalassaemia major, careful echocardiographic measurements have been made over a period of several years. A similar approach has been used by Henry *et al.*[29] However, two difficulties arise in studying the groups. First, the individuals in the groups are growing children, and absolute increases in dimensions may be attributable to a normal growing process or to a pathological chamber dilatation. Secondly, the population is anaemic and this may lead to either acute or chronic dimensional changes. Chronic anaemia leads to an increase of resting cardiac output and stroke volume, particularly when haemoglobin levels are below 7 g/100 ml. In general, the haemoglobin is maintained at rather higher levels in our population of thalassaemic children. With regard to the acute effects of transfusion, we have not demonstrated any consistent echocardiographic changes in dimensions measured just prior to and following transfusions. Before chelation therapy is commenced, there is a direct relationship between left ventricular internal diastolic diameter and the number of units of blood transfused and, to a lesser degree, with age. This is believed to represent impaired systolic function due to iron overload. The ejection fraction appears a less sensitive index of ventricular function. These findings are in broad agreement with those of other series[29] using a slightly more diverse patient population. In order to eliminate the effects of varying body sizes of the children, the ventricular dimensions can be expressed as a 'standard deviation score', which is the number of standard deviations from the normal for the body surface area. Serial measurements from our own series have indicated a number of patients undergoing chelation therapy in whom there has been a progressive reduction of the standard deviation score, implying that the ventricular function is returning towards normality. Some isolated variations occur; one child died of rapidly progressive heart failure without marked ventricular dilatation. To date we have not demonstrated that any other conventional echocardiographic measurement or derivative to be a more sensitive indicator of early myocardial damage. In the limited number of patients with echocardiograms before and after transfusion, we have not found this subacute cardiac stress to isolate any cases who may have incipient heart failure. We have not seen the deterioration associated with ascorbic acid supplement described in an American series.

Radionuclide angiography may be used as an alternative method of monitoring changes of ventricular function. At rest some patients with haemochromatosis demonstrated a reduced ejection fraction[30] and, for this degree of ventricular abnormality, the echocardiographic assessment of ejection fraction is probably as sensitive as radionuclide angiography. Earlier degrees of cardiac damage may be demonstrated by repeating the angiography after exercise.[20,28] Patients receiving less than 100 units of blood show no significant differences from controls in the resting ejection fraction and, in all cases examined, a normal increase occurred on exercise. With greater iron loading, the ejection fraction generally falls on exercise and amongst this group are all the cases with clearly abnormal resting angiograms. The effect of chelation therapy on this pattern of response has yet to be shown. Both series reported to date have shown isolated cases with focal abnormalities of wall motion without any clear underlying mechanism. The abrupt deterioration in cardiac function which seems to occur when haemochromatosis leads to heart failure has suggested that when a critical toxic level of iron develops, then serious myocardial cell impairment occurs. While moderate iron loading clearly has no detectable cardiac effect, the longer term studies on transfusional haemochromatosis suggest that progressive iron loading leads to progressive myocardial depression. The use of echocardiographic and radionuclide measurements of ventricular function to follow the long-term course in a significant size of population of idiopathic haemochromatosis has not been reported. My experience of a limited number of such patients is that the resting echocardiogram is frequently normal in the absence of overt cardiac dysfunction and that some form of stress test would be required to pick up early changes.

Treatment of the iron-loaded heart centres on methods of removing the stored iron, either by venesection or by chelating agents. The former generally takes 1–2 years to deplete all the excess iron in idiopathic forms. However, the severely ill patient with heart failure requires careful management of the fluid status using diuretics and, if appropriate, venesection. The generalized nature of the disease must not be overlooked during this stage, particularly the diabetic and hepatic features. Arrhythmias should be treated with conventional methods although ventricular tachycardias may become very resistant to drugs.

In summary, it is clear that iron overload, of whatever cause, leads to myocardial damage. There is a long latent period of diffuse iron accumulation. ECG changes and arrhythmias may mark definite cardiac involvement. Alternatively, subtle changes in left ventricular function may be demonstrated by echocardiography or radionuclide angiography. Eventually congestive heart failure develops, occasionally with a restrictive pattern and, if untreated, the prognosis is limited to 1–2 years. There is encouraging evidence that the process is reversible, even at a late stage, although treatment needs to be continued for 1–2 years to remove most of the iron. The mechanism of the myocardial failure remains unclear and further studies on the early stages are needed to determine progression of changes during the late period. For the cardiologist, haemochromatosis should be considered in any case presenting as a cardiomyopathy. For other specialists, cardiac involvement should be sought in any patient known to have, or known to be at risk of, iron overload.

ACKNOWLEDGEMENT

I am grateful to Dr. D. M. Flynn of the Royal Free Hospital for the very considerable help he has given and the opportunity to study his patients with thalassaemia major.

REFERENCES

1. Powell LW, Halliday JW. The liver and iron storage disease. In: Powell LW, ed. *Metals and the liver*. New York: Dekker, 1978.
2. Williams R, Pitcher CS, Parsonson A, William HS. Iron absorption in the relatives of patients with idiopathic haemochromatosis. *Lancet* 1965; **1**: 1243.

3. Beaumont C, Simon M, Fauchet R et al. Serum ferritin as a possible marker of the haemochromatosis allele. *N Engl J Med* 1979; **301**: 169.
4. Alarcon PA, Donovan M, Forbes G, Landaw SA, Stockman JA. Iron absorption in the thalassaemia syndromes and its inhibition by tea. *N Engl J Med* 1979; **300**: 5.
5. Williams R, Smith PM, Spicer EJF, Barry M, Sherlock S. Venesection therapy in idiopathic haemochromatosis. *Q J Med* 1969; **38**: 1.
6. Barry M, Flynn DM, Letsky EA, Ridson RA. Long term chelation therapy in thalassaemia major: effect on liver iron concentration, liver histology and clinical progress. *Br Med J* 1974; **2**: 16.
7. Peters TJ, Seymour CA. Acid hydrolase activities and lysosomal integrity in liver biopsies from patients with iron overload. *Clin Sci Mol Med* 1976; **50**: 75.
8. Lewis HP. Cardiac involvement in haemochromatosis. *Am J Med Sci* 1954; **227**: 554.
9. Finch SC, Finch CA. Idiopathic haemochromatosis, an iron storage disease. *Medicine (Balt)* 1955; **34**: 381.
10. Powell LW. Changing concepts in haemochromatosis. *Postgrad Med J* 1970; **46**: 200.
11. Bomford A, Williams R. Long term results of venesection therapy in idiopathic haemochromatosis. *Q J Med* 1976; **45**: 611.
12. Mattheyses M, Hespel JP, Brissot P et al. La myocardiopathie de l'hemochromatose idiopathique. *Arch Mal Coeur Vaisseaux* 1978; **71**: 371.
13. Short EH, Winkle RA, Billingham ME. Myocardial involvement in idiopathic haemochromatosis. *Am J Med* 1981; **70**: 1275.
14. Easley RM, Schreiner BF, Yu PN. Reversible cardiomyopathy associated with haemochromatosis. *N Engl J Med* 1972; **287**: 866.
15. Skinner C, Kenmure ACF. Haemochromatosis presenting as congestive cardiomyopathy and responding to venesection. *Br Heart J* 1973; **35**: 466.
16. Wasserman AJ, Richardson EW, Baird CL, Wyso EM. Cardiac haemochromatosis simulating constrictive pericarditis. *Am J Med* 1962; **32**: 316.
17. Nody AC, Bruno MS, De Pasquale NP, Bienstock PA. Fulminating idiopathic haemochromatosis simulating constrictive pericarditis. *Ann Intern Med* 1975; **83**: 373.
18. Cutler DC, Isner JM, Bracy AW et al. Haemochromatosis heart disease: an unemphasized cause of potentially reversible restrictive cardiomyopathy. *Am J Med* 1980; **69**: 923.
19. Tyberg TI, Goodyer AVN, Hurst VW, Alexander J, Langou RA. Left ventricular filling in differentiating restrictive cardiomyopathy and constrictive pericarditis. *Am J Cardiol* 1981; **47**: 791.
20. Leon MB, Borer JS, Bacharach SL et al. Detection of early cardiac dysfunction in patients with severe beta thalassaemia and chronic iron overload. *N Engl J Med* 1979; **301**: 1143.
21. Engle MA, Erlandson M, Smith CH. Late cardiac complications of chronic severe refractory anaemia with haemochromatosis. *Circulation* 1964; **30**: 698.
22. Feely J, Counihan TB. Haemochromatosis presenting as angina and responding to venesection. *Br Med J* 1977; **2**: 681.
23. Slama R, Motte G, Coumel P et al. Les blocs auriculoventriculaires de l'hemochromatose. *Nouv Presse Med* 1979; **79**: 747.
24. Arnett EN, Nienhuis AW, Henry WL et al. Massive myocardial haemosiderosis: a structure-function conference at the National Heart and Lung Institute. *Am Heart J* 1975; **90**: 777.
25. Vigorita VJ, Hutchins GM. Cardiac conduction system in haemochromatosis: clinical and pathological features of six patients. *Am J Cardiol* 1979; **44**: 418.
26. Buja ML, Roberts WC. Iron in the heart. *Am J Med* 1971; **51**: 209.
27. Fitchett DH, Coltart DJ, Littler WA et al. Cardiac involvement in secondary haemochromatosis: a catheter biopsy study and analysis of myocardium. *Cardiovasc Res* 1980; **14**: 719.

28. Nienhuis AW, Benz EJ, Propper R et al. Thalassaemia major: molecular and clinical aspects. *Ann Intern Med* 1979; **91**: 883.
29. Henry WC, Nienhuis AW, Wiener M, Miller DR, Canale VC, Piomelli S. Echocardiographic abnormalities in patients with transfusion-dependent anaemia and secondary myocardial iron deposition. *Am J Med* 1978; **64**: 547.
30. Hellenbrand WE, Berger HJ, O'Brien RT, Talner NS, Zaret BL. Left ventricular performance in thalassaemia—a combined non-invasive radionucleide and echocardiographic assessment. *Circulation* 1977; **55**: and **56**: Suppl. III, 49.

Chapter 5

Cardiac abnormalities associated with hereditary neuromuscular diseases

Tom Evans

FRIEDREICH'S ATAXIA

Introduction

This is a rare spinocerebellar neuromyelopathy usually transmitted as an autosomal recessive.[1] Typically there is an early onset of progressive ataxia, dysarthria, posterior column signs in the lower limbs and muscle weakness.[2,3] Friedreich[4] found cardiac involvement at autopsy in his original description of this syndrome and both Ormerod[5] and Newton Pitt[6] noted ante-mortem clinical cardiac failure. Although many patients die from heart failure[7,8] overt cardiac signs and symptoms tend to be manifest late in the natural history of the disease.[9,10] Several authors have stressed that bedside clinical evaluation is difficult because auscultatory abnormalities are infrequent,[9–12] heart size on the chest radiograph is difficult to evaluate because of the scoliosis[2,11] and electrocardiographic changes, although usual, are non-specific.[12–14]

Hewer[7] reviewed the clinical records of 82 fatal cases of Friedreich's ataxia and noted that 73 per cent of the patients had cardiac symptoms prior to death. In 12 of the 22 patients who did not have cardiac symptoms the ECG was normal in only 2. Hewer suggested that the heart is probably always abnormal in true Friedreich's ataxia, pointing out that the ECG is abnormal in 90 per cent of cases and there were no published reports of a normal heart being found at autopsy. A further feature noted by this author in the same paper was that atrial fibrillation occurred in many cases and often appeared to precipitate cardiac failure. The loss of atrial systole in patients with hypertrophic cardiomyopathy[15,16] may result in acute cardiac decompensation probably due to the abnormal diastolic function of the left ventricle,[17] increasing the importance of atrial transport. As the heart muscle disease described by various authors[18–25] may functionally resemble hypertrophic cardiomyopathy with or without obstruction, Hewer's observation is of especial interest.

Pathology

Sanchez-Casis et al.[26] extensively reviewed the literature relating to the observed pathology of the heart in Friedreich's ataxia and concluded that:

1. Macroscopically there was consistent cardiac dilatation with some degree of ventricular hypertrophy and mild atrial dilatation.
2. Microscopically the more important and constant histological changes were myocardial fibrosis and degeneration of myocardial cells. Granular deposits of calcium and iron were found in the myocardial cells.
3. Cardiac disease resembling hypertrophic cardiomyopathy, occasionally with outflow tract obstruction, appeared to be an integral part of Friedreich's ataxia. However, myofibrillar disarray, considered by some cardiac pathologists[27,28] to be an essential feature of the histology of true hypertrophic cardiomyopathy, had never been recorded. This latter fact, together with the echocardiographic studies[25] which will be quoted later, suggests that although left ventricular hypertrophy occurs in Friedreich's ataxia it may be incorrect to identify it too exactly with the 'idiopathic' by definition cardiomyopathy.[29]

Electrocardiographic Features

Mollaret[13] and Rathery et al.[30] reported ECG abnormalities but Evans and Wright[12] described the first large ECG series; 30 per cent of 38 patients had ST–T changes and they observed one case of complete heart block. Boyer,[11] in a series of 31 patients, noted ST–T changes in 16 patients and atrial arrhythmias in 3. Thoren[31] found only 3 out of 49 patients had normal resting ECGs and concluded that in the most severely affected patients with Friedreich's ataxia, atrial tachyarrhythmias, right axis deviation and right ventricular hypertrophy predominated. ST–T changes of varying degree were present in 41 of the 49 patients. Thoren concurred with Evans,[12] finding that similar ECG abnormalities might occur in affected members of the same family.

Gregorini et al.[32] demonstrated abnormal vectorcardiograms compatible with diffuse myocardial damage in 10 patients. In 5 of those patients the 12 lead ECG was normal. Malo et al.,[14] reviewing their experience in the Quebec Cooperative Study of Friedreich's ataxia, recorded both normal ECG and VCG findings in only 1 patient out of

35. They postulated that the VCG was more explicit in demonstrating the severity of the QRS changes, with a right ventricular hypertrophy pattern present in 60 per cent. In this series 4 ECGs and 3 VCGs were normal. This prevalence of RVH is both surprising and difficult to explain. Indeed in this latter series 2 patients with ECG and VCG changes of RVH who were studied by cardiac catheterization had haemodynamically significant left ventricular outflow tract obstruction, gradients of 78 and 60 mm Hg respectively. Catheter studies in another patient showed right ventricular outflow tract obstruction but most series do not suggest that this is a common finding. The effect of scoliosis on the ECG and VCG should not be ignored but does not explain the findings.

Echocardiographic Findings

In the Quebec Cooperative Study[24] 21 patients aged from 7 to 28 years underwent echocardiographic study; 90 per cent of studies were considered to be abnormal. The results may be summarized as follows:

Septal hypertrophy	81 per cent
Left ventricular free wall hypertrophy	61 per cent
Slight reduction of left ventricular internal dimension	57 per cent
Asymmetrical septal hypertrophy	29 per cent
Systolic anterior motion of the mitral valve	3 patients
Symmetrical left ventricular hypertrophy and left ventricular enlargement	2 patients

A previous echocardiographic study by Smith[10] showed asymmetrical septal hypertrophy in 4 patients, septum/posterior wall ratio ranging from 1·4 to 1·9, mean 1·66 (normal $<1{\cdot}3$).

St. John Sutton et al.[25] studied 7 patients using computer-assisted analysis of the left ventricular echocardiograms and compared the findings with those of 45 normal children matched for age and sex. They concluded that 'the absence of asymmetric septal hypertrophy and mid systolic closure of the aortic valve, the presence of normal septal motion and the greater reduction in posterior wall than in septal dynamics are inconsistent with previous ideas that the heart disease of Friedreich's ataxia is identical to hypertrophic cardiomyopathy'.

Haemodynamic and Angiographic Studies

The most comprehensive studies were those undertaken in the Quebec Study (Cote et al.[33] and Guerin et al.[34]). Previous studies[18–21,23,35] had indicated that left ventricular hypertrophy, with or without asymmetrical septal hypertrophy and with or without outflow tract obstruction, could occur. Ruschhaupt[21] had reported a case in whom a presumptive diagnosis of hypertrophic obstructive cardiomyopathy was made some years prior to the neurological presentation. The Quebec Study confirmed that the heart muscle disease associated with Friedreich's ataxia usually takes the form of concentric left ventricular hypertrophy but asymmetrical, even obstructive, hypertrophy can occur. In a small number of patients a diffusely hypokinetic left ventricle was found.

Summary

Heart muscle disease appears to be an intrinsic part of the syndrome of Friedreich's ataxia, especially in the advanced stages. The functional and morphological picture in many patients is that of concentric left ventricular hypertrophy, although a picture resembling in some respects hypertrophic obstructive cardiomyopathy is well recognized.

DUCHENNE'S MUSCULAR DYSTROPHY

Muscular dystrophies have been defined as a group of genetically determined disorders with progressive destruction of skeletal muscle in the absence of any associated structural abnormality of either the central or the peripheral nervous systems.[36] They have been subdivided into various types on the basis of the clinical distribution, the severity of muscle weakness and the pattern of inheritance. Cardiac involvement is most frequently seen in the so-called 'Duchenne' variety. Duchenne published his first paper on 'paraplegie hypertrophie' in 1861[37] and by 1868[38] had collected data on 13 cases of paralysie musculaire pseudohypertrophique. In the latter report he described pre-mortem muscle biopsy to confirm the diagnosis and this is almost certainly why the eponym 'Duchenne' has remained although Dr. Edward Meryon probably described the clinical details of the first affected family in 1851.[39] Early case reports are well reviewed by Accardo.[40] The Duchenne syndrome has an incidence of 1 in 3–4000 male births, being inherited as a sex-linked recessive.[41] The age of onset is usually between 18 months and 5 years.[42] By 11 years of age most boys are unable to walk, and death, sometimes sudden, frequently occurs between 14 and 21 years. Becker[43] described a variant with a similar muscle group distribution to that of the Duchenne form but often associated with a relatively benign prognosis. The uncles of affected males were often found to be aged 30–50 years and neurological examination revealed only mild to moderate disability. Cardiac involvement appears to be rare in this variant and in most other forms of muscular dystrophy.[44]

Cardiac disease in Duchenne's dystrophy has been reported by many authors, but the exact incidence has varied, probably depending upon the neurological criteria used and the age group studied. Ross[45] first described myocardial atrophy in a 12-year-old boy with pseudohypertrophic dystrophy and by 1923 Globus,[46] in reporting a further case, was able to review another 10 cases from the literature; Globus suggested that the histological changes seen in the myocardium were, in fact, the cardiac manifestations of systemic dystrophy. Subsequent reports, however, have demonstrated that the myocardial changes are similar to those seen in skeletal muscle, although less diffuse, and were present in all patients at necropsy.[42,47–53]

Myocardial involvement is undoubtedly very common in this syndrome although it is uncertain at what age or stage of the disease it begins. Electrocardiographic changes are often present in very young patients, inferring early involvement of the heart.[42] Various authors have failed to demonstrate any correlation between the degree of skeletal muscle disease, the severity of cardiac symptoms and ECG abnormalities. ECG abnormalities are also seen in some female carriers of the disease with serum enzyme abnormalities.[54]

Pathology

Cardiac histology in reported series shows fatty and fibrous tissue replacement of the myocardium with selective scarring of the posterolateral wall of the left ventricle which sometimes involves the posterior papillary muscle. The large epicardial coronary arteries are normal, although James[56] has described non-inflammatory small arterial disease. However, Perloff[57] has pointed out that the distribution of scarring is unrelated to this 'arteriopathy'. A high incidence of mitral valve prolapse has been documented in this syndrome, although mitral valve prolapse is perhaps such a common finding in the general population for this to be arguably a chance association. Sanyal[58] performed two necropsy examinations of the hearts of children who had died from classical Duchenne dystrophy and had had mitral valve prolapse documented ante-mortem. The main abnormality demonstrated was fibrosis and myofibrillolysis—most extensive in the posterior papillary muscles and the posterobasal segments of the left ventricles when matched with control hearts. The mitral valve annulus, its leaflets and the origin, distribution pattern, length and thickness of the chordae tendineae were entirely normal. These autopsy studies correlate well with those of Perloff and may help explain the almost specific ECG pattern in patients with this syndrome.

Clinical Findings

Persistent or labile sinus tachycardia is a frequent finding. This was first noted by Meerwein,[59] and Boas and Lowenberg[60] emphasized that the sleeping heart rate tended to be rapid and to accelerate further in response to minor stimuli. Perloff[61] has suggested that the traditional explanation of the tachycardia being a manifestation of the 'immobilization syndrome' is incorrect and that augmented sympathetic activity is present. There are no other specific clinical findings in Duchenne dystrophy. Overt cardiac failure is rare as the patients are frequently immobile but some echocardiographic and haemodynamic studies to be referred to later suggest that left ventricular function is impaired in varying degrees.

The Electrocardiogram

Perloff has pointed out that although several neurological disorders may be associated with abnormal electrocardiograms, only one, the Duchenne moiety, produces a distinct almost diagnostic trace.[57] The vectorcardiogram is a useful supplement to the 12 lead ECG.[62]

Typical ECG changes have been reported by many authors in 50–90 per cent of cases.[42,57,61] The changes are tall R waves across the right praecordium with increased R/S amplitude ratios; deep Q waves in the limb leads and over the left lateral praecordium. At times the deep Q waves occur together with altered shapes of right praecordium R waves (RSr′ or polyphasic r waves). Siblings with the syndrome tend to have quite similar tracings and, as previously mentioned, female carriers may have abnormal ECGs.

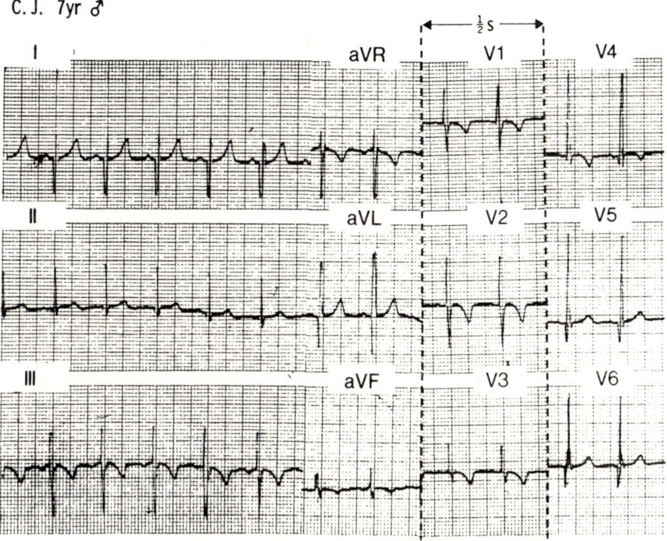

Figure 1. ECG from a 7-year-old child with Duchenne's muscular dystrophy (courtesy of Dr. Katherine Hallidie-Smith).

The mechanism of the characteristic electrocardiographic changes is debatable. Perloff points out that studies performed so far make it clear that the specific ECG changes are *not* related to thoracic deformity, thoracic muscle atrophy or pulmonary hypertension. Neither are they related to hypertrophy of the right ventricle, crista supraventricularis, interventricular septum or to abnormalities in the right ventricular outflow tract or co-existing abnormalities of the small intramural coronary arteries. Perloff favours the theory that ECG abnormalities reflect acquired dystrophic myocardial disease, the sites of which are genetically regulated, rather than the theory which proposes that the morphology of the ECG represents a genetically determined persistence of the patterns of infancy and early childhood.[63] The fact that the ECGs of siblings with classical Duchenne dystrophy tend to be identical would perhaps suggest that the disease may·be almost unique in genetically 'labelling' a specific portion of left ventricular myocardium to be affected—Kovick's study[66] demonstrating impairment of posterior wall movement suggests this hypothesis, as do the necropsy studies of Perloff,[57] Rubler[65] and Sanyal.[58] In the necropsy studies of Perloff[57] and Rubler,[65] precise mapping of the ventricles and interventricular septum demonstrated selective transmural scarring of the postero-basal left ventricle, with or without lateral or inferior wall extension, suggesting acceptable electrocardiographic/vectorcardiographic/necropsy correlations.[67]

Echocardiographic Studies

Kovick et al.[66] examined posterior left ventricular wall motion in 3 patients aged 15, 16 and 22. They found a reduced maximal diastolic endocardial velocity and postulated that these results reflected impaired myocardial relaxation produced by dystrophic heart disease.

Ahmad et al.[68] studied 13 children echocardiographically and digitized the parameters of left ventricular function to facilitate computer analysis. All systolic indices were considered normal but the maximal diastolic endocardial velocity was reduced, confirming Kovick's report. No other indices were significantly different from control and it was concluded that myocardial function was well-preserved in children with the Duchenne syndrome. Ahmad suggested that the reduced maximal endocardial velocity could be the result of reduced overall movement of the heart within the thorax. Heymsfield[69] noted evidence of depressed left ventricular function usually in the later stages of the disease. Vincent[70] used echocardiography to examine left ventricular posterior wall thickness in nine patients with the Duchenne dystrophy and characteristically prominent anterior in lead VI of the electrocardiogram. He found end-diastolic left ventricular wall thickness to be diminished in these patients and felt that this strongly supported the previously outlined concepts of Perloff regarding the genesis of the ECG. Reeves,[71] however, did not find any evidence of reduced posterior wall thickness.

Mitral valve prolapse was found in 11 out of 20 patients studied prospectively by Sanyal[72] whereas Reeves[71] found an incidence of 25 per cent.

Taken together, Perloff's hypothesis of a focal lesion of the posterior wall and papillary muscle area appears to have significant if not conclusive combined ECG, ECHO and necropsy support.

Haemodynamic Studies

Relatively few haemodynamic studies have been performed in patients with Duchenne's dystrophy. Most of the studies have been confined to the right side of the heart[73] and there has been a suggestion that latent left ventricular failure may be precipitated by exercise in some patients. Demany[74] reported a case in whom intractable cardiac failure was associated with the haemodynamic and left ventricular ciné-angiographic appearances of severe left ventricular failure. Interestingly the patient had had recurrent supraventricular arrhythmias, and coronary angiography showed an abrupt ending of the artery to the sino-atrial node, this latter finding being later confirmed at autopsy.

BECKER'S DYSTROPHY AND LIMB GIRDLE DYSTROPHY OF ERB

This is much rarer than the Duchenne variety, but Katiyar[75] has described a family in whom heart muscle disease appeared in one member, whilst the other neurologically affected members were spared. It can be difficult to distinguish some forms of Becker type dystrophy from the limb-girdle type dystrophy described by Erb, especially if accurate family trees are not available. In some of these cases patients thought to have the Becker type of dystrophy have demonstrated the cardiac problems seen in Erb's syndrome. These are infrequent and not usually severe, invariably consisting of atrial arrhythmias and conduction defects at all levels. Rarely a combination of conducting system disease and ventricular dysfunction have been observed in sporadic cases of Erb's dystrophy.[76,77]

FACIO-SCAPULOHUMERAL DYSTROPHY (LANDOUZY–DEJERINE SYNDROME)

The course of this disease is long and insidious with a far better prognosis than in most other forms of muscular dystrophy. However, very rare cases of conducting system disease and congestive cardiac failure have been described,[78] as has electromechanical atrial paralysis[79] perhaps similar to that occurring in the humeroperoneal syndrome.

DYSTROPHIA MYOTONIA

Steinert[80] described this autosomal dominant disorder which characteristically presents in the third or fourth decades of life, although younger patients are described.

The clinical picture is usually typical with myotonia that can be produced by voluntary, mechanical or electrical stimulation of the hands, forearms, tongue and jaw. The dystrophic element initially presents in the forearms, the neck muscles, particularly the sternocleidomastoids, and as expressionless facies. Cataracts, gonadal atrophy, frontal baldness or thinning of the hair are usually associated, and gastrointestinal muscle problems have been described.

Griffith[81] drew attention to the sinus bradycardia occurring in dystrophia myotonia. However, Adie and Greenfield[82] described 20 cases and as they found that in 1 case examined at autopsy the heart was grossly normal and in another the electrocardiogram was normal, they felt it was unlikely that the heart was usually affected in this syndrome. Maas and Zondek,[83] Guillain and Rouques,[84] Mondon and Pasquet[85] and Carrillo[86] all described cases with ECG abnormalities, mainly sinus bradycardia or a prolonged PR interval—Segura and Lawari,[87] however, described 11 patients with no cardiac abnormalities. Evans[88] reviewed the literature and 13 personal cases. A prolonged PR interval was present in 6 cases with QRS notching in 10 cases. Cardiomegaly tended to be associated with bradycardia. One of Evans' cases had intermittent 2:1 atrio-ventricular block.

Spillane[89] and Fisch[90] reviewed the subject extensively, the latter author concluding that, of 85 cases of dystrophia myotonia, 68 per cent had abnormal electrocardiograms and that, of these, 91 per cent were conduction defects and/or arrhythmias. Litchfield[91] reported a case, seemingly unique at that time, in which the presentation was with Adams–Stokes attacks, during one of which the patient succumbed. The patient had demonstrated electrocardiograms with sinus bradycardia, complete heart block and alternating left and right bundle branch blocks. Ephedrine hydrochloride was unsuccessful in controlling the attacks and undoubtedly this 42-year-old woman died of a cardiac arrhythmia.

More recent studies confirm that clinical evidence of cardiac involvement is common in dystrophia myotonia occurring in approximately two-thirds of patients.[92–94] The electrocardiogram is frequently abnormal, as previously indicated, but overt clinical evidence of heart muscle disease is rare, being present in only approximately 7 per cent of patients. Interestingly, the disease may present as cardiac disease before the neuromuscular syndrome becomes apparent.

The most common ECG finding is sinus bradycardia with prolongation of the PR interval. Sino-atrial disease of the bradycardia/tachycardia variety has been observed. Infra-Hisian blocks are usually abnormalities of conduction in the left bundle branch and include left anterior hemiblock. Rate-dependent left bundle branch block, which later becomes permanent, has been described. Cardiac arrhythmias, particularly atrial, may also occur.

Studies using His-bundle electrocardiography have located the conduction disturbance to the His–Purkinje system in most cases.[95] A prolonged conduction in this system is recognized as a frequent precursor of atrio-ventricular block. Prystowsky et al.[96] studied nine patients with dystrophia myotonia by performing several electrophysiological studies in an attempt to predict whether those patients at greatest risk of complete block and sudden death could be identified with a view to permanent pacemaker implantation.

Nine patients were evaluated at a mean time of 35 months apart. At the initial study 7 patients had first-degree atrio-ventricular block and 3 of the 7 patients had evidence of His–Purkinje conduction delay (HV 55 msec). At the time of the second study 7 patients had prolonged HV intervals and over the 3-year period of the study, HV intervals increased by a least 5 msec in all 7 patients. No electrophysiological or electrocardiographic parameters could be found that correlated with progression of the conduction disturbance in these patients. In conclusion, Prystowsky et al. recommended invasive studies only for symptomatic patients. It seems reasonable to suggest, however, that perhaps 24-hour ambulatory monitoring might be considered to screen for serious conduction disturbances. Insertion of permanent transvenous pacemaking systems is mandatory if syncope or severe bradycardia occurs.

As well as the conduction disorders previously discussed, low voltage P waves, ST segment abnormalities and flattening or inversion of T waves are common. Rarely an electrocardiographic pattern resembling myocardial infarction has been described.

Frequently cardiomegaly, if present, is asymptomatic but frank congestive cardiac failure may be provoked or aggravated by inappropriately slow heart rates.

Reviewing the pathology of the myocardium, it has become obvious that although histological abnormalities of the myocardium sometimes occur, they appear to be in no way analogous to the dystrophic disease that affects the skeletal muscle.[97]

The significant incidence of sudden cardiac death in dystrophia myotonia should never be overlooked as many patients will cope for many years with their skeletal muscle problems, making the insertion of a permanent pacemaker system both justifiable and rewarding. The cardiac conduction defects that occur in this disease make the use of phenytoin, which does not depress cardiac conduction, a much safer alternative to procainamide, which is a powerful depressant of the cardiac conducting system—although both drugs have beneficial effects in the treatment of the skeletal muscle disorder.

SCAPULOPERONEAL SYNDROME

This X-linked scapuloperoneal syndrome differs from the X-linked humeroperoneal syndrome in its clinical presentation. It has been described by several groups of workers[98–100] and the incidence of complete heart block, permanent pacemaker implantation and even sudden death is quite high. The myopathy may be very subtle and many patients are seemingly at greater risk of dying from cardiac arrhythmia than other problems. Hassan et al.[100] described a 31-year-old man who had been serving in the army for 8 years until the age of 28 years. He had found that he could not pick up a load when he was kneeling down but when standing could lift a load of 100 lb. On neurological examination he had only a subtle scapular and peroneal myopathy but there was electrocardiographic evidence of sino-atrial and atrio-ventricular disease. An extensive examination of a known pedigree of 101 family members revealed 12 males with skeletal muscle involvement and 6 of these required permanent pacemaker implantation by the age of 30 years, for marked bradycardia.

Various ECG findings have included sinus arrest with junctional rhythms, infranodal atrio-ventricular blocks (His–Purkinje disease) and both atrial flutter and fibrillation.

Intracardiac electrophysiological studies have revealed prolonged HV times and recording from the right atrium reveals no atrial potential, nor does the atrium respond to electrical stimulation.

There appears to be no relationship between atrial arrhythmias, supra- and infra-Hisian blocks and the severity of the skeletal muscle disease—nor does the left ventricular function appear to be compromised.

CHARCOT–MARIE–TOOTH DISEASE (PERONEAL MUSCULAR ATROPHY)

This autosomal dominant disease almost invariably affects the cardiac conducting system rather than the ventricular myocardium. Both the sick sinus syndrome and complete atrio-ventricular block are well documented. Littler[101] described a family in which 10 members of 3 generations were affected. Three patients had both peroneal muscular atrophy and conduction defects, 6 patients had various conduction defects including RBBB and 1 patient had the neurological syndrome alone.

HUMEROPERONEAL DYSTROPHY

This syndrome is characterized by peroneal and humeral muscular weakness with contractures developing in the first decade of life and stabilizing near the end of the second decade.[102]

Cardiac involvement usually takes the form of atrial arrhythmias, atrial electromechanical paralysis and bradycardias. Junctional rhythms with complete heart block (infra-nodal) or infra-Hisian blocks are recognized.

Whether it is a completely discrete entity from the scapuloperoneal syndrome is unclear.

REFERENCES

1. Andermann E, Remillard GM, Goyer C et al. Genetic and family studies in Friedreich's ataxia. *Can J Neurol Sci* 1976; **3**: 287–301.
2. Geoffroy G, Barbeau A, Breton G et al. Clinical description and roentgenologic evaluation of patients with Friedreich's ataxia. *Can J Neurol Sci* 1976; **3**: 279–86.
3. Walton JN. *Brain's diseases of the nervous system*. New York: Oxford University Press, 1977: 672.
4. Friedreich N. Über degenerative atropie der spinalen Hinterstränge. *Arch Pathol Anat* 1863; **26**: 391 and 433.
5. Ormerod JA. On the so-called hereditary ataxia, first described by Friedreich. *Brain* 1885; **7**: 105–31.
6. Pitt GN. On a case of Friedreich disease. Its clinical history and postmortem appearances. *Guy's Hosp Rep* 1886–87; **44**: 369.
7. Hewer RL. Study of fatal cases of Friedreich's ataxia. *Br Med J* 1968; **2**: 649–52.
8. Van der Hauwert LG, Dunmoulin M. Hypertrophic cardiomyopathy in Friedreich's ataxia. *Br Heart J* 1976; **38**: 1291–8.
9. Cote M, Davignon A, Pecko-Drouin K et al. Cardiological signs and symptoms in Friedreich's ataxia. *Can J Neurol Sci* 1976; **3**: 319–21.
10. Smith ER, Sangalang VE, Heffernan LP, Welsh JP, Flemington CS. Hypertrophic cardiomyopathy: the heart disease of Friedreich's ataxia. *Am Heart J* 1977; **94**: 428–34.
11. Boyer SH IV, Chisholm AW, McKusick VA. Cardiac aspects of Friedreich's ataxia. *Circulation* 1962; **25**: 493–505.
12. Evans W, Wright G. The electrocardiogram in Friedreich's ataxia. *Br Heart J* 1942; **4**: 91–102.
13. Mollaret P. *La maladie de Friedreich*. Thèse de Paris. 1929.
14. Malo S, Latour Y, Cote M, Geoffroy G, Lemieux B, Barbeau A. Electrocardiographic and vectorcardiographic findings in Friedreich's ataxia. *Can J Neurol Sci* 1976; **3**: 323–8.
15. Goodwin JF. Prospects and predictions for the cardiomyopathies. *Circulation* 1974; **50**: 210.

16. Evans TR. Heart muscle disease. *Medicine* 1979; series 3: 1042–7.
17. Sanderson JE, Traill TA, St. John Sutton MG, Brown DJ, Gibson DG, Goodwin JF. Left ventricular relaxation and filling in hypertrophic cardiomyopathy. An echocardiographic study. *Br Heart J* 1978; **40**: 596–601.
18. Boehm TM, Dickerson RB, Glasser SP. Hypertrophic subaortic stenosis occurring in a patient with Friedreich's ataxia. *Am J Med Sci* 1970; **260**: 279–84.
19. Gach JV, Andriange M, Franck G. Hypertrophic obstructive cardiomyopathy and Friedreich's ataxia. Report of a case and review of literature. *Am J Cardiol* 1971; **27**: 436–41.
20. Elias G, Guerin R, Spitaels Fouron JC, Davignon A. Sténose musculaire sous-aortique et ataxie de Friedreich. *Union Med Can* 1972; **101**: 474–8.
21. Ruschhaupt DG, Thilenius OG, Cassels DE. Friedreich's ataxia with idiopathic hypertrophic subarotic stenosis. *Am Heart J* 1972; **84**: 95–102.
22. Olsen EG. Cardiomyopathies. *Cardiovasc Clin* 1972; **4**: 239–51.
23. Gabriel B, Pinsard N, Gerard R, Louchet E. Association d'une cardiomyopathie et d'une dégénérescence spino-cérébelleuse (maladie de Friedreich): à propos d'une observation. *Pediatrie* 1974; **29**: 367–77.
24. Gattiker HF, Davignon A, Bozio A et al. Echocardiographic findings in Friedreich's ataxia. *Can J Neurol Sci* 1976; **3**: 329–32.
25. St. John Sutton MG, Olukotun AY, Tajik AJ, Lovett JL, Giulani ER. Left ventricular function in Friedreich's ataxia. An echocardiographic study. *Br Heart J* 1980; **44**: 309–16.
26. Sanchez-Casis, Cote M, Barbeau A. Pathology of the heart in Friedreich's ataxia: review of the literature and report of one case. *Can J Neurol Sci* 1976; **3**: 349–54.
27. Maron BJ, Savage DD, Clark CE et al. Prevalence and characteristics of disproportionate ventricula septal thickening in patients with coronary artery disease. *Circulation* 1978; **57**: 250.
28. Olsen EGJ. Endomyocardial biopsy. Editorial. *Br Heart J* 1978; **40**: 95–8.
29. Brandenburg RO, Chazov E, Cherian G et at. Report of the WHO/ISFG Task Force on definition and classification of cardiomyopathies. *Circulation* 1981; **64**: 437–38A.
30. Rathery F, Mollaret P, Stern J. *Bull Mem Soc Med Hôp Paris* 1934; **50**: 1382.
31. Thoren C. Cardiomyopathy in Friedreich's ataxia. *Acta Paediatr Scand* 1964; supplement 153.
32. Gregorini L, Valentini R, Libretti A. The vectorcardiogram in Friedreich's ataxia. *Am Heart J* 1974; **87**: 158–63.
33. Cote M, Davignon A, Elias G et al. Haemodynamic findings in Friedreich's ataxia. *Can J Neurol Sci* 1976; **3**(4): 319–21.
34. Guerin R, Elias G, Davignon A et al. Cardiac angiographic findings in Friedreich's ataxia. *Can J Neurol Sci* 1976; **3**(4): 337–42.
35. Ivemark B, Thoren G. The pathology of the heart in Friedreich's ataxia. *Acta Med Scand* 1964; **175**: 227.
36. Walton JN. In: *Brain's diseases of the nervous system.* New York, Toronto, London: Oxford University Press, 1977: 8th ed: 995.
37. Duchenne de Boulogne GBA. *De l'electrisation localisée et de son application à la pathologie et à la thérapeutique.* Paris: Ballière, 1861.
38. Duchenne de Boulogne GBA. Recherches sur la paralysie musculaire pseudo-hypertrophique, on paralysie myo-sclérosique. *Arch Gen Med* 1868; **11**: 5–25, 179–209, 305–21, 421–43, 552–88.
(Selections translated in Wilkins RH, IA, eds. *Neurological classics.* New York: Johnson Reprint, 1973: 59–67.)
39. Meryon E. On granular and fatty degeneration of the voluntary muscles. *Med Chir Trans* 1852; **35**: 73–84.
40. Accardo PJ. An early case report of muscular dystrophy: a footnote to the history of neuromuscular disorders. *Arch Neurol* 1981; **38**: 144–6.

41. Walton JN. The inheritance of muscular dystrophy: further observations. *Ann Hum Genet* 1956; **21**: 40.
42. Dubowitz V. *Muscle disorders in children.* London, Philadelphia: Saunders, 1978.
43. Becker PE, Kiener F. Eine neue X-chromosomale Muskeldystrophie. *Arch Psychiat Nervenkr* 1955; **193**: 427.
44. Perloff JK. Neurological disorders and heart disease. In: Braunwald E, ed. *Heart disease.* Philadelphia, London, Toronto: Saunders, 1981.
45. Ross J. On a case of pseudohypertrophic paralysis. *Br Med J* 1883; **1**: 200–2.
46. Globus JH. The pathologic findings in the heart muscle in progressive muscular dystrophy. *Arch Neurol Psychiat (Chic)* 1923; **9**: 59–72.
47. Bevans M. Changes in the musculature of the gastrointestinal tract and in the myocardium in progressive muscular dystrophy. *Arch Pathol* 1945; **40**: 225–38.
48. Moore WF Jr. Cardiac involvement in progressive muscular dystrophy. *J. Paediatr* 1954; **44**: 683–7.
49. Schott J, Jacobi M, Wald MA. Electrocardiographic patterns in the differential diagnosis of progressive muscular dystrophy. *Am J Med Sci* 1955; **229**: 517–24.
50. Watson H. *Paediatric cardiology.* London: Lloyd-Luke, 1968: 770.
51. Dubowitz V. *Progressive muscular dystrophy in childhood.* University of Cape Town: Thesis, 1960.
52. Rubin IL, Buchberg AS. The heart in progressive muscular dystrophy. *Am Heart J* 1952; **43**: 161–9.
53. Berenbaum AA, Horowitz W. Heart involvement in progressive muscular dystrophy. Report of a case with sudden death. *Am Heart J* 1956; **51**: 622–7.
54. Mann O, de Leon AC, Perloff JK, Simawis J, Horrigan FD. Duchenne's muscular dystrophy. The electrocardiogram in female relatives. *Am J Med Sci* 1968; **59**: 255–376.
55. Emery AEH. Abnormalities of the electrocardiogram in female carriers of Duchenne muscular dystrophy. *Br Med J* 1969; **2**: 418–20.
56. James TN. Observations on the cardiovascular involvement, including the cardiac conduction system, in progressive muscular dystrophy. *Am Heart J* 1962; **63**: 48.
57. Perloff JK, Roberts WC, de Leon AC, O'Dohert D. The distinctive electrocardiogram of Duchenne's progressive muscular dystrophy. *Am J. Med* 1967; **42**: 179.
58. Sanyal KS, Johnson WW, Dische MR, Pitner SE, Beard C. Dystrophic degeneration of papillary muscle and ventricular myocardium. A basis for mitral valve prolapse in Duchenne's muscular dystrophy. *Circulation* 1980; **62**: 436–7.
59. Meerwin H. *Verhaltnisse von Hertz und Zunge bei den primaren myopathien.* Basel: Dissertation, 1904.
60. Boas EP, Lowenberg H. Heart rate in progressive muscular dystrophy. *Arch Intern Med* 1931; **47**: 376.
61. Perloff JK. The myocardial disease of heredofamilial neuromyopathies. In: Fowler N, ed. *Myocardial disease.* New York: Grune & Stratton, 1973.
62. Fitch CW, Ainger LE. The Frank vectorcardiogram and the electrocardiogram in Duchenne muscular dystrophy. *Circulation* 1976; **35**: 1124.
63. Slucka C. The electrocardiogram in Duchenne's progressive muscular dystrophy. *Circulation* 1968; **38**: 933.
64. Skyring A, McKusick VA. Clinical, genetic and electrocardiographic studies in childhood muscular dystrophy. *Am J Med Sci* 1961; **242**: 54.
65. Rubler S, Perloff JK, Roberts WC. Clinical pathological conference—Duchenne's muscular dystrophy. *Am Heart J* 1977; **94**: 776.
66. Kovick RB, Fogelman AM, Abbasi AS, Peter JB, Pearce ML. Echocardiographic evaluation of posterior left ventricular wall movement in muscular dystrophy. *Circulation* 1975; **52**: 447.
67. Perloff JK. Neurological disorders and heart disease. In: Braunwald E, ed. *Heart disease.* Philadelphia, London, Toronto: Saunders, 1981.

68. Ahmad M, Sanderson JE, Dubowitz V, Hallidie-Smith KA. Echocardiographic assessment of left ventricular function in Duchenne's muscular dystrophy. *Br Heart J* 1978; **40**: 734–40.
69. Heymsfield SB, McNish T, Perkins JV, Felner JM. Sequence of cardiac changes in Duchenne's muscular dystrophy. *Am Heart J* 1978; **95**: 283.
70. Vincent GM, Davis D, Ziter F. Echocardiography in Duchenne dystrophy. *Circulation* 1975; **52**: suppl. 2: 78.
71. Reeves WC, Griggs R, Nanda WC, Thomson K, Gramiak R. Echocardiographic evaluation of cardiac abnormalities in Duchenne's dystrophy and myotonic muscular dystrophy. *Arch Neurol* 1980; **37**: 5.
72. Sanyal SK, Leung R, Tierney RC, Gilmartin R, Pitner SE. Mitral valve prolapse syndrome in Duchenne's progressive muscular dystrophy. *Paediatrics* 1979; **83**: 116.
73. Rubeiz GA, Saab NG. Hemodynamic study in a case of progressive muscular dystrophy involving the heart. *Am J Cardiol* 1962; **10**: 890.
74. Demany MA, Zimmerman HA. Progressive muscular dystrophy: haemodynamic, angiographic and pathologic study of a patient with myocardial involvement. *Circulation* 1969; **40**: 377–84.
75. Katiyar BC, Misia S, Somani PN, Chaterji AM. Congestive cardiomyopathy in a family of Becker's X-linked muscular dystrophy. *Postgrad Med J* 1977; **53**: 12.
76. Lambert CD, Fairfax AJ. Neurological associations of chronic heart block. *J Neurol Neurosurg Psychiatr* 1976; **39**: 571.
77. Fairfax AJ, Lambert CD. Neurological aspects of sinoatrial heart block. *J. Neurol Neurosurg Psychiatr* 1976; **39**: 576.
78. Gailani S, Danowski TS, Fisher DS. Muscular dystrophy: catheterization studies indicating latent congestive heart failure. *Circulation* 1958; **17**: 583.
79. Baldwin AJ, Talley RC, Johnson C, Nutter DO. Permanent paralysis of the atrium in a patient with facioscapulohumeral muscular dystrophy. *Am J Cardiol* 1973; **31**: 649.
80. Steinert H. Myopathologische Beitrage. I. Ueber das klinische und anatomische Bild des Muskelschwunds der Myotoniker. *Dtsch Z Nervenheilk* 1909; **37**: 58.
81. Griffith TW. On myotonia. *Q J Med* 1911–1912; **5**: 229.
82. Adie WJ, Greenfield JG. Dystrophia myotonica (myotonia atrophica). *Brain* 1923; **46**: 73.
83. Maas O, Zondek H. *Z Neurol Psychiatr* 1920; **59**: 322.
84. Guillain G, Rouquès L. Le coeur dans la myotone atrophique. *Ann Med (Paris)* 1932; **31**: 158.
85. Mondon H, Pasquet D. Le coeur dans la myotonie atrophique. *Arch Mal Coeur* 1939; **32**: 401.
86. Carillo EG. El electrocardiograma en la distrofia muscular familiar. *Rev Argent Cardiol* 1941; **8**: 122.
87. Segura RG, Lawari A. El aparato cardiovascular en los sindromes miotonicos. *Rev Argent Cardiol* 1941; **7**: 363.
88. Evans W. The heart in myotonia atrophica. *Br Heart J* 1944; **6**: 41.
89. Spillane JD. The heart in myotonia atrophica. *Br Heart J* 1941; **13**: 343.
90. Fisch C. The heart in dystrophia myotonica. *Am Heart J* 1951; **41**: 525.
91. Litchfield JA. A–V dissociation in dystrophia myotonica. *Br Heart J* 1953; **15**: 357.
92. Holt JM, Lambert EHN. Heart disease as the presenting feature in myotonia atrophica. *Br Heart J* 1964; **26**: 433.
93. Petkovich NJ, Dunn M, Reed W. Myotonia dystrophica with A–V dissociation and Stokes–Adams attacks. *Am Heart J* 1964; **68**: 391.
94. Clements SD, Colmers RA, Hurst JW. Ventricular arrythmias, intraventricular conduction abnormalities, atrioventricular block and Stokes–Adams attacks successfully treated with permanent transvenous pacemaker. *Am J Cardiol* 1976; **37**: 93.

95. Josephson ME, Caracta AR, Gallagher JJ, Damato AN. Site of conduction disturbances in a family with myotonic dystrophy. *Am J Cardiol* 1973; **32**: 114.
96. Prystowsky EN, Pritchett ELC, Roses AD, Gallagher J. The natural history of conduction system disease in myotonic muscular dystrophy as determined by serial electrophysiological studies. *Circulation* 1979; **60** (6): 1360–9.
97. Vemura N, Tanaka H, Miimura T et al. Electrophysiological and histological abnormalities of the heart in myotonic dystrophy. *Am Heart J* 1973; **86**: 616.
98. Thomas PK, Calne DR, Elliott CF. X-linked scapuloperoneal syndrome. *J Neurol Neurosurg Psychiatr* 1972; **35**: 208.
99. Thomas PK, Schott GD, Morgan-Hughes JA. Adult onset scapuloperoneal myopathy. *J. Neurol Neurosurg Psychiatr* 1975; **38**: 1008.
100. Hassan ZU, Fastabend CP, Mohanty PK, Isaacs ER. Atrioventricular block and supraventricular arrhythmias with X-linked muscular dystrophy. *Circulation* 1979; **60** (6): 1365–9.
101. Littler WA. Heart block and peroneal muscular atrophy. *Q J Med* 1970; **39**: 431.
102. Waters DD, Nutter DO, Hopkins LC, Dorney ER. Cardiac features of an unusual X-linked humeroperoneal muscular disease. *N Engl J Med* 1975; **293**: 1017.

Chapter 6

Acromegalic heart disease

John S. Jenkins

INTRODUCTION

Cardiac enlargement has been recognized as a feature of acromegaly since the end of the nineteenth century[1] soon after the disease was first described by Pierre Marie in 1886. An increase in cardiac mass has frequently been found at autopsy[2-4] and sometimes this enlargement is of an extreme degree. *Figure 1* shows the heart from a woman aged 55, who died in heart failure, and who had suffered from acromegaly for at least 7 years. She also had hypertension, the blood pressure being initially 170/120, which was subsequently controlled with methyldopa. Nevertheless, the enormous weight of the heart, 1021 g, appeared to be quite excessive for this degree of hypertension.

Cardiac enlargement in acromegaly has been ascribed to a variety of factors, particularly hypertension, coronary artery disease and diabetes, but cardiac abnormalities are undoubtedly found in some patients who have none of these complications. It has been suggested that cardiac hypertrophy could occur as a direct result of the increased secretion of growth hormone,[3,5] although others[6] have denied the existence of a specific acromegalic cardiomyopathy.

Wright et al.[7] published a detailed survey of mortality in patients with acromegaly and showed that the death rate for patients aged 45–65 with the disease was twice that of the unaffected population. When the nature of the deaths was analysed, cardiovascular causes were most prominent, amounting to 24 per cent, although in this retrospective investigation no detailed assessment of the extent to which hypertension was a factor could be made in the individual patients.

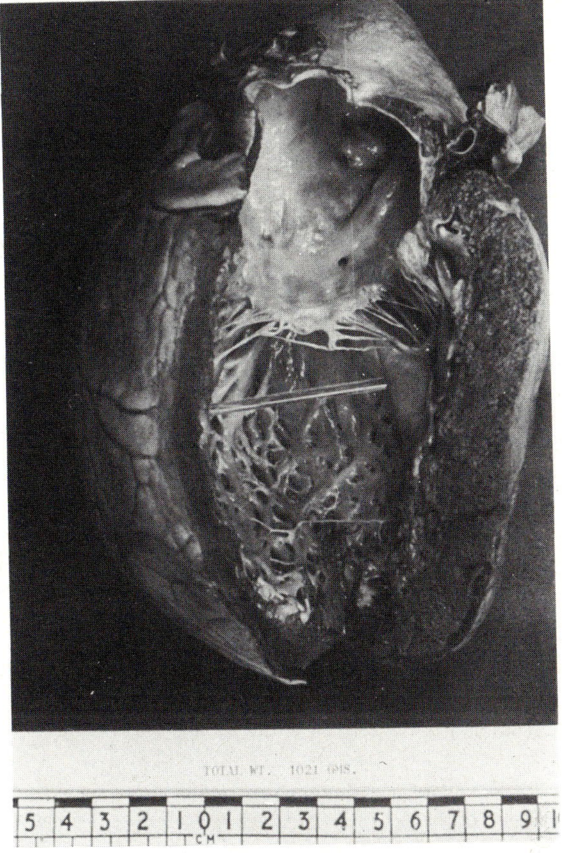

Figure 1. Heart from woman aged 55 who had suffered from acromegaly for 7 years.

CLINICAL STUDIES

Echocardiographic Changes in Acromegaly

In order to study the increase in cardiac size during life, its relationship to hypertension, and the cardiac performance, 24 acromegalic patients were investigated using echocardiography and systolic time interval measurements.[8] Their ages ranged from 24 to 80 years; 4 were untreated, and the remainder had received either radiotherapy or pituitary surgery up to 9 years previously (Table 1). Seven patients (29 per cent) had hypertension, an incidence which is similar to that of other series,[6,9] although only 3 patients had a diastolic pressure over

Table 1
Clinical details of patients with acromegaly

Patient	*Age (years)*	*Sex*	*Blood pressure (mm Hg)*	*Estimated duration of disease (years)*	*Time since treatment (years)*	*Growth hormone (mu/L)*	
						Initial	*Current*
1	24	F	130/80	8	5	—	5·2
2	24	F	140/80	11	6	300	7·0
3	27	F	120/70	2	1	20	4·8
4	28	F	120/80	9	8	340	2·4
5	48	F	160/115	13	8	76	9·0
6	49	F	140/90	4	3	114	4·8
7	53	F	120/80	1	—	176	176
8	57	F	220/110	16	1	125	1·0
9	58	F	140/90	7	2	24	5·6
10	59	F	140/110	9	6	11	1·8
11	67	F	135/90	10	7	60	5·5
12	27	M	120/80	10	6	26	1·2
13	28	M	140/80	14	—	420	420
14	36	M	140/90	4	2	200	2·2
15	37	M	120/80	10	9	44	4·5
16	41	M	120/80	2	1	60	1·9
17	46	M	120/80	12	3	100	1·3
18	49	M	120/85	10	3	37	3·1
19	51	M	135/100	12	3	12	2·2
20	55	M	130/90	8	5	290	18
21	56	M	150/100	30	—	30	30
22	57	M	150/95	27	5	61	5·2
23	80	M	190/110	6	4	34	14
24	53	M	140/90	18	—	150	150
Normal						<5	

100 mm Hg. The duration of the disease was estimated to range from 1 to 18 years. Only 1 patient had diabetes mellitus and 1 had suffered from a myocardial infarction 1 year previously. None of the other patients had a history of ischaemic heart disease and none had clinical evidence of heart failure. The initial plasma growth hormone concentrations before treatment varied greatly and treatment resulted in normal values being restored in 13 out of 20 patients.

Left Ventricular Mass

From the echocardiographic measurements 14 patients (58 per cent) had a left ventricular mass greater than 200 g but only 4 of these had hypertension (Table 2). In fact the three highest values were found in the normotensive group (*Figure 2*), and the largest left ventricle of all the series, 780 g, was present in an apparently fit 28-year-old man without hypertension, who had suffered from acromegaly for about 14

Table 2
Echocardiographic and systolic time interval measurements and calculations

Patient	*Posterior wall thickness (PWT) (cm)*	*Inter-ventricular septal thickness (IST) (cm)*	*IST/PWT ratio*	*Left ventricular mass (g)*	*Ejection fraction*	*PEP/LVET ratio*
1	0·8	1·0	1·25	249	0·75	0·31
2	0·9	0·9	1·0	227	0·70	0·38
3	0·85	0·8	0·94	134	0·66	0·41
4	0·8	0·75	0·94	173	0·71	0·41
5	1·2	1·3	1·08	221	0·78	0·39
6	1·0	1·25	1·25	288	0·70	0·41
7	0·6	0·50	0·83	158	0·41	0·80
8	1·0	0·95	0·95	138	0·72	0·33
9	1·5	2·0	1·33	583	0·66	0·38
10	0·8	1·5	1·88	246	0·76	0·31
11	0·85	0·9	1·06	173	0·66	0·35
12	1·0	0·7	0·7	134	0·69	0·38
13	1·5	1·4	0·93	788	0·69	0·41
14	1·0	0·95	0·95	277	0·73	0·37
15	0·7	0·8	1·14	189	0·70	0·37
16	0·75	0·7	0·93	116	0·68	0·42
17	1·2	1·6	1·33	489	0·70	0·33
18	1·0	1·2	1·2	213	0·71	0·42
19	0·85	0·9	1·06	174	0·69	0·39
20	0·95	1·7	1·79	321	0·70	0·63
21	0·9	0·8	0·89	136	0·84	0·39
22	1·05	1·3	1·24	272	0·66	0·52
23	1·05	1·0	0·95	372	0·68	0·53
24	1·0	1·7	1·7	327	0·78	—
Normal subjects Mean	0·7*	0·8*	< 1·3	140*	0·75*	0·35*
SD	0·1	0·1		30	0·07	0·04
Range	0·5–0·9	0·6–1·0		80–200	0·61–0·89	0·27–0·4

* Values obtained from 20 normal subjects (10 male and 10 female) aged 24–54 years (mean 39 years).

years (Table 2, Patient 13). There was no definite correlation between the left ventricular mass and the magnitude of the growth hormone concentration or the duration of the disease. Similar results have been obtained by other investigators using echocardiography.[9, 10]

Interventricular Septal Hypertrophy

It has been reported that there is a particularly high incidence of asymmetric septal hypertrophy in acromegalic hearts.[11] In 5 patients

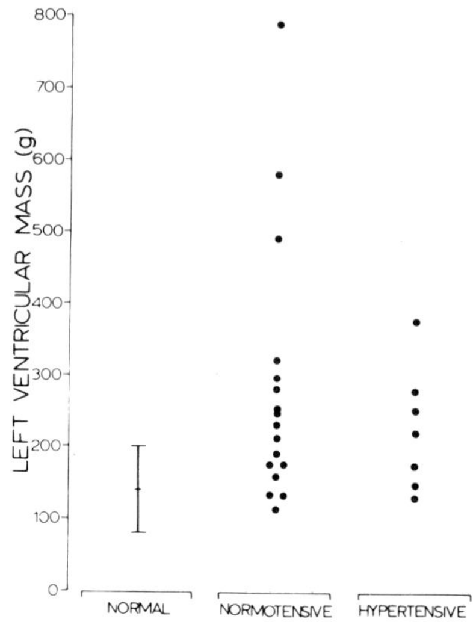

Figure 2. Left ventricular mass (LVM) in normotensive and hypertensive acromegalic patients compared with the normal range.

from the present series the septum was disproportionately thick (Table 2, Patients 9, 10, 17, 20, 24), but the septum–posterior ventricular wall ratio was considerably increased in only 3 patients, of whom 1 was hypertensive. In this series the frequency of asymmetric septal hypertrophy was no greater than that reported in other types of cardiac hypertrophy,[12] and this abnormality is not a special feature of acromegaly.

Left Ventricular Function

An important part of the investigation was to determine to what extent acromegaly was associated with a deterioration in cardiac function. Cardiac failure has been frequently reported in patients with acromegaly,[2,3,5] but even in the absence of gross signs of heart failure it has been suggested that there is a high incidence of subclinical myocardial dysfunction.[13]

Left ventricular function was assessed using both the ejection fraction obtained from echocardiographic measurements, and the pre-ejection period–left ventricular ejection time (PEP/LVET) ratio derived from the phonocardiograph, carotid pulse tracing, and ECG (Table 2 and *Figure 3*). The PEP/LVET ratio was abnormal in 4 patients only, of whom 1 had already suffered from a myocardial infarction (Tables 1 and 2, Patient 20), 1 was of extreme age (Patient 23), and 1 had co-

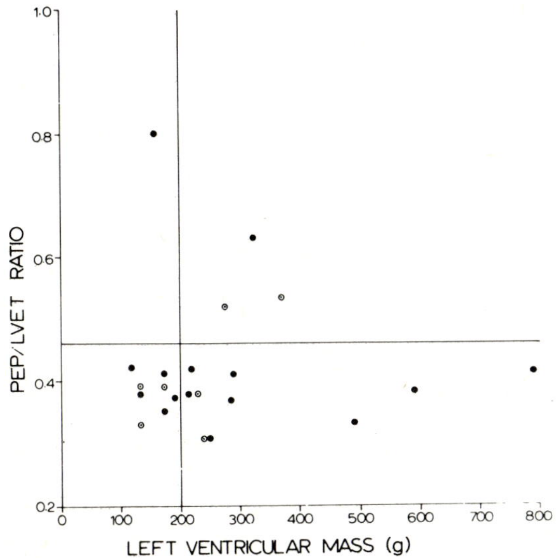

Figure 3. Relation between pre-ejection period/left ventricular ejection time (PEP/LVET) ratio and left ventricular mass.

existent Addison's disease (Patient 7). Despite the fact that the adrenocortical insufficiency in this patient had been treated for many years with adequate hormone therapy its contribution to cardiac performance was difficult to assess. Only 1 patient, therefore, had an otherwise unexplained abnormal PEP/LVET ratio. *Figure 3* shows that there was no relationship to left ventricular mass; the three largest hearts apparently functioned normally.

There is now considerable evidence that the ejection fraction provides the best overall index of basal left ventricular function.[14] Table 2 shows that only Patient 7, with Addison's disease, had an abnormal ejection fraction. There is, therefore, no evidence that left ventricular dysfunction is common in patients with acromegaly, even in the presence of considerable ventricular hypertrophy, and these findings are in accordance with other published studies.[9,10]

It is, however, uncertain to what extent cardiac function of individual patients may deteriorate in the future, since there is experimental evidence that cardiac hypertrophy induced by various stimuli will lead to diminishing contractility of the muscle, and ultimately to heart failure. It was important, therefore, to determine whether regression of cardiac size could occur after removal of the excessive growth hormone secretion.

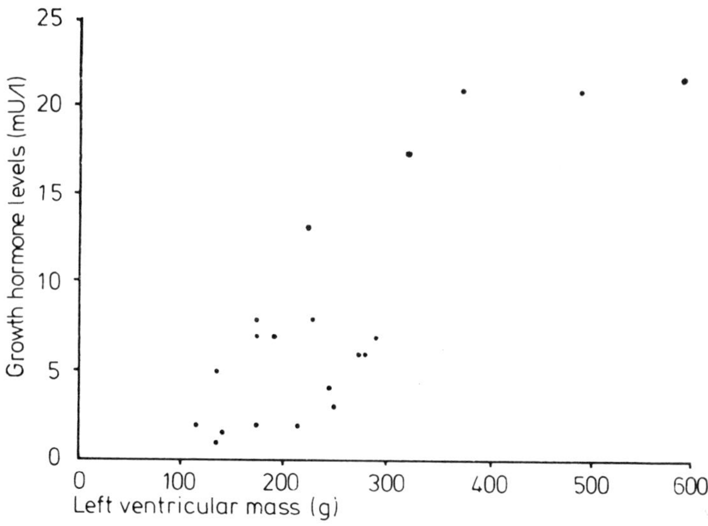

Figure 4. Relation between left ventricular mass and growth hormone levels achieved after treatment of acromegalic patients (Mather et al.[8]).

Left Ventricular Mass after Treatment of Acromegaly

In the 20 treated patients the degree of left ventricular enlargement was plotted against the mean plasma growth hormone concentration achieved during the 12 months previous to the study (*Figure 4*). Generally, left ventricular mass was normal or only moderately increased in patients whose growth hormone values had been within the normal range for the previous year, whereas cardiac hypertrophy was much greater in those patients whose treatment had been unsuccessful or in whom reduction of growth hormone was very recent. These observations are not conclusive but they suggest that some reversal of cardiac enlargement is possible after effective treatment. A definitive answer to this important question will, however, require serial use of echocardiography.

ANIMAL STUDIES

In order to investigate more directly the effects of excessive growth hormone secretion on the heart an animal model was developed.[14] Much of the previous work in this field has been carried out by injecting growth hormone into hypophysectomized animals for relatively short periods of time,[15,16] but these studies have not been very satisfactory, firstly because enough species-specific growth hormone has not been available for prolonged experiments, and secondly because the intermittent dosage given does not really reproduce the clinical state of acromegaly. There is, however, a rat pituitary tumour cell line, designated GH_3, which secretes large amounts of growth hormone, and which can be cultured *in vitro*.[17] When a suspension of these cells was inoculated subcutaneously into the Wistar–Furth strain of rat a palpable tumour appeared after about 6 weeks, which then continued to secrete large amounts of growth hormone. It is thus possible to produce 'acromegalic' rats (*Figure 5*). Over a period of 11 weeks a linear increase in body weight occurred when compared with control rats (*Figure 6*), so that at the end of this time the body weight doubled and the tail to nose length was 30 per cent greater. The mean plasma growth hormone concentration was considerably increased, being

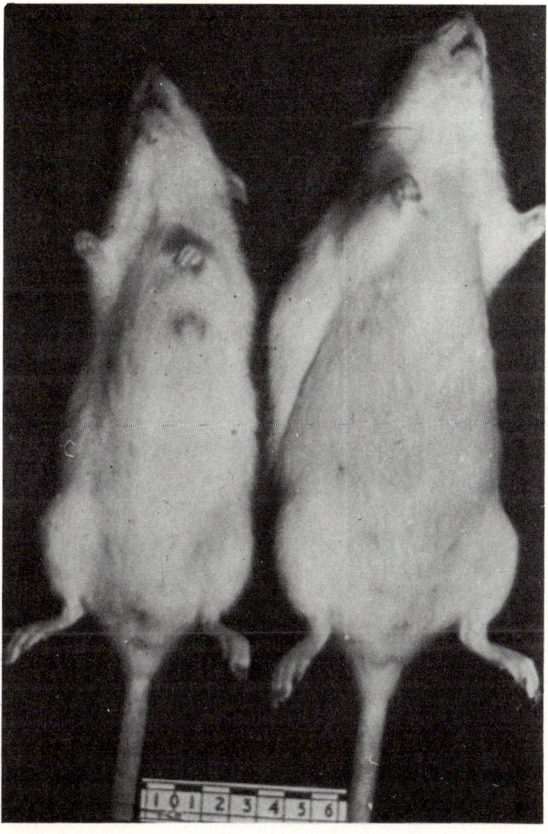

Figure 5. Normal rat and animal bearing a growth hormone-secreting tumour.

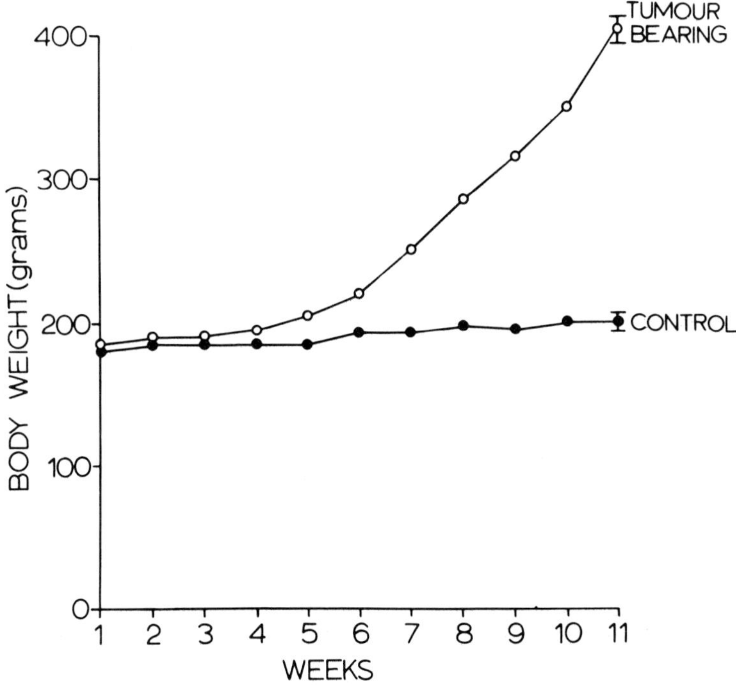

Figure. 6. Total body weight of normal animals (●) and of rats bearing growth hormone-secreting tumours (○). Standard error bars are shown for animals at the time of death (Prysor-Jones and Jenkins[14]).

2500 μg/l in all animals with tumours, compared with values for control rats of 60 ± 9 SEM μg/l. There was no increase in the blood pressure, and blood glucose levels remained normal so that none of the animals became diabetic.

The Heart and Other Viscera in Tumour-bearing Rats

Table 3 shows that in rats bearing growth hormone-secreting tumours the heart weight was increased 138 per cent above control values, skeletal muscle less so, but kidney, liver and spleen were increased to an even greater extent than the heart. A recent report on the pathological changes in 27 acromegalic patients at autopsy[4] described very similar changes although, not surprisingly, they were less uniform than those seen in the experimental animals. Nevertheless, the increases in heart size of the patients ranged up to 270 per cent above the expected normal weight and there were considerable increases in the size of the liver, spleen and kidneys. Histological examination of the rat 'acro-

Table 3
Body and organ weights in normal, and tumour-bearing rats secreting growth hormone (values are means ± S.E.M.)

Parameter measured	*Normal*	*Tumour-bearing*	*Weight increase (% control)*
Body (g)	200·2 ± 5·6	409·0 ± 9·6	105
Liver (g)	6·4 ± 0·4	22·6 ± 0·6	253
Kidney (g)	1·3 ± 0·1	3·6 ± 0·1	161
Spleen (mg)	356·0 ± 10·9	1306·0 ± 44·1	267
Heart (mg)	640·3 = 21·7	1526·0 ± 33·8	138
Tibialis anterior (mg)	423·4 ± 21·0	593·4 ± 24·7	40
Rectus femoris (mg)	645·0 ± 33·4	871·0 ± 36·3	35
Vastus lateralis (mg)	611·5 ± 37·2	835·0 ± 42·6	37

megalic' heart showed hypertrophy of the muscle fibres but there were none of the additional changes found by Lie and Grossman[4] in the human myocardium such as interstitial fibrosis and lymphomononuclear infiltrates. It is not certain whether these histological variations are related to species differences or to a very different time scale for exposure to growth hormone. The increase in cardiac muscle bulk is to be explained by hypertrophy of the fibres and is generally considered to be due to increased protein synthesis of the myocardium. There have been previous studies showing that growth hormone stimulates protein synthesis both in cardiac and skeletal muscle,[18] but there is no information on the effect of the hormone on DNA synthesis in the myocardium.

Effects of Excessive Growth Hormone Secretion on DNA Synthesis of Heart and Skeletal Muscle

[^{3}H]-thymidine was administered to rats with and without tumours 2 hours before death and its incorporation into DNA extracted from cardiac and skeletal muscle was measured (Table 4). In the presence of

Table 4
Incorporation of [^{3}H]-thymidine into DNA of heart and skeletal muscle (d.p.m./μg) (values are means ± S.E.M.)

Organ	*Normal rats*	*Tumour-bearing rats*	*Increase (% control)*	*P value*
Heart	12·5 ± 4·0	53·4 ± 4·7	327	<0·005
Vastus lateralis	4·4 ± 0·7	13·9 ± 2·3	216	<0·02
Soleus	5·0 ± 1·0	17·8 ± 2·4	256	<0·01

excessive growth hormone secretion DNA synthesis in heart muscle was over four times, and in skeletal muscle was over three times, that of control animals. Zak[19] has shown that there is increased myocardial DNA synthesis after cardiac hypertrophy has been induced in the rat by aortic constriction. This increase is ascribed to both polyploidy of myocardial cell nuclei as well as an increase in the extramyocardial connective tissue. Autoradiography of the histological section of myocardium in the 'acromegalic' rat showed that the tritium label was in the myocardial cell nuclei. At least in the rat, therefore, growth hormone stimulates DNA of cardiac muscle cell nuclei as well as increasing muscle bulk by protein synthesis.

Effect of Removal of Excessive Growth Hormone on Size of Heart and Other Viscera

The experimental animal model provided a direct means by which regression of cardiac mass could be studied after removal of the excessive growth hormone secretion. After tumours had been induced in rats the animals were divided into two groups, from one of which the tumours were surgically removed and the animals were allowed to recover. Eight weeks after plasma growth hormone concentrations had returned to normal the animals were killed and the organ weights were compared with those of animals retaining their tumours, and with normal animals (*Figure 7*). During this period of time the size of the

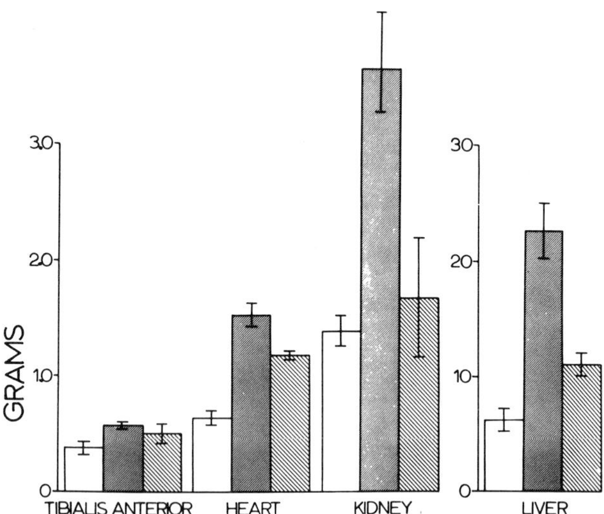

Figure 7. Weight of heart and other organs of rats bearing tumours (shaded bars) compared with animals from which tumours had been removed (hatched bars) and normal control animals (open bars). Each bar is the mean ± S.E.M. (Prysor-Jones and Jenkins[14]).

heart did not return to normal but was reduced by 25 per cent compared with the tumour-bearing animals. In the case of other organs, especially liver and kidney, the reduction in size was even greater.

CONCLUSIONS

These studies show that, irrespective of hypertension, excessive growth hormone secretion is associated with an increase in cardiac mass both in the clinical condition of acromegaly and in the experimental animal.

In the case of the rat, at least, the cardiac muscle fibre hypertrophy induced by growth hormone is accompanied by an increase in DNA synthesis. Despite an increase in left ventricular mass, which in some patients may occur to an extreme degree, impaired left ventricular function in acromegaly is not common. It should be emphasized, however, that the long-term effects of cardiomegaly in individual patients are not yet known, although previous mortality studies have undoubtedly shown an increased number of cardiac deaths in older patients with acromegaly. With the advent of echocardiography the serial study of patients during life has become possible and this will undoubtedly give more information on the progression of acromegalic heart disease. It seems likely that a combination of factors is responsible for the final outcome—specific growth hormone-induced hypertrophy, coronary artery disease and, in some patients, hypertension. Clinical evidence suggests, and the experimental findings show more clearly, that some regression of cardiac size can occur if growth hormone secretion is restored to normal. These observations provide a further incentive to treat acromegaly as actively as possible.

ACKNOWLEDGEMENTS

I am grateful to the Editor of the *British Heart Journal* for permission to reproduce *Figure 4* and to the *Journal of Endocrinology* for *Figures 6* and 7.

REFERENCES

1. Huchard H. Anatomie pathologique, lésions et troubles cardio-vasculaires de l'acromegalie. *J Practiciens* 1895; **9**: 249.
2. Hejtmancik MR, Bradfield JY, Hermann GR. Acromegaly and the heart: a clinical and pathological study. *Ann Intern Med* 1951; **34**: 1445–56.
3. Courville CB, Mason VR. The heart in acromegaly. *Arch Intern Med* 1938; **61**: 704–13.
4. Lie JT, Grossman SJ. Pathology of the heart in acromegaly: anatomic findings in 27 autopsied patients. *Am Heart J* 1980; **100**: 41–52.
5. Pepine CJ, Aloia J. Heart muscle disease in acromegaly. *Am J Med* 1970; **48**: 530–4.

6. McGuffin W L, Sherman BM, Roth J et al. Acromegaly and cardiovascular disorders. *Ann Intern Med* 1974; **81**: 11–18.
7. Wright AD, Hill DM, Lowy C, Fraser TR. Mortality in acromegaly. *Q J Med* 1970; **39**: 1–16.
8. Mather HM, Boyd MJ, Jenkins JS. Heart size and function in acromegaly. *Br Heart J* 1979; **41**: 697–701.
9. Martins JB, Kerber RE, Sherman BM, Marcus ML, Ehrhardt JC. Cardiac size and function in acromegaly. *Circulation* 1977; **56**: 863–9.
10. Savage DD, Henry WL, Eastman RC, Borer JS, Gorden P. Echocardiographic assessment of cardiac anatomy and function in acromegalic patients. *Am J Med* 1979; **67**: 823–9.
11. Hearne MJ, Sherber HS, de Leon AC. Asymmetric septal hypertrophy in acromegaly—an echocardiographic study. (Abstract.) *Circulation* 1975: **51**, **52**; Suppl. II: 35.
12. Maron BJ, Clark CE, Henry WL. et al. Prevalence and characteristics of disproportionate ventricular septal thickening in patients with acquired or congenital heart diseases. *Circulation* 1977; **55**: 489–96.
13. Jonas EA, Aloia JF, Lane FJ. Evidence of subclinical heart muscle dysfunction in acromegaly. *Chest* 1975 **67**: 190–4.
14. Prysor-Jones RA, Jenkins JS. Effect of excessive secretion of growth hormone on tissues of the rat with particular reference to the heart and skeletal muscle. *J. Endocrinol* 1980; **85**: 75–82.
15. De Grandpré R, Raab W. Interrelated hormonal factors in cardiac hypertrophy: experiments in non-hypertensive hypophysectomized rats. *Circ Res* 1953; **1**: 345–53.
16. Bates RW, Milkovic S, Garrison MM. Effects of prolactin, growth hormone, and ACTH, alone and in combination upon organ weights and adrenal function in normal rats. *Endocrinology* 1964; **74**: 714–23.
17. Tashjian AH, Yasumura Y, Levine L, Sato G, Parker ML. Establishment of clonal strains of rat pituitary tumour cells that secrete growth hormone. *Endocrinology* 1968: **82**, 342–52.
18. Kostyo JL, Nutting DF. Growth hormone and protein metabolism. In: Knobil E, Sawyer WH, eds. *Handbook of physiology, endocrinology. The pituitary gland and its neuroendocrine control.* Sect. 7, vol. IV, pt 2, ch. 29. Washington DC: American Physiological Society, 1974: 187–210.
19. Zak R. Development and proliferative capacity of cardiac muscle cells. *Circ Res* 1974; **35**: suppl. II: 17–26.

Chapter 7

Thyroid heart disease

Cecil Symons

INTRODUCTION

Caleb Parry in 1786 was the first to describe hyperthyroidism and it is of specific interest that his attention was drawn to this condition by cardiac symptoms and signs occurring in a young woman who later developed a goitre and weight loss; the cardiac manifestations preceded the overt endocrine disturbance, emphasizing from the outset of the first description of hyperthyroidism, the important association of thyroid and heart disease. Over-activity of the thyroid gland manifests itself by an increase in cardiac work, however defined, and it has always been a matter for argument whether or not there is any permanent adverse effect on the heart. Whatever the answer, there is no doubt that marked and occasionally serious cardiotoxic effects are produced concurrently with thyroid disease which usually, but not always, disappear once the endocrine condition is controlled.

In light of current awareness of heart muscle disease, it is fair to state that the subtle effects which may occur in the heart muscle are of no less importance than the long recognized cardiac arrhythmias and even coronary disease. In fact, these phenomena merge with each other and any rigid attempt to delineate one from another can produce an artificial separation. This chapter will therefore survey both the immediate and long-term changes that may arise in all varieties of thyroid heart disease.

Laboratory investigation using increasingly sophisticated tests will produce earlier diagnosis of thyroid disorder but all too frequently the physician, endocrinologist or cardiologist will not think speedily enough of the underlying endocrine abnormality in his patient with unexplained cardiac illness. Such is the ease of application of thyroid function tests that there is justification for the use of screening investigations in any form of cardiac disorder which presents obscure features in diagnosis, e.g. in specific heart muscle disease, idiopathic atrial fibrillation or even sino-atrial disease. Additionally, both the clinician and physiologist may see in thyroid disease how marked alteration in the circulatory state affects the basically healthy heart and, should some other pathological cardiac condition be already present, how this is affected by a disturbed metabolic or mechanical load. Insufficient attention has probably been given to the availability of this almost physiological model, for thyroid disease will increase or diminish every known response of the heart in health or disease. Severe thyroid problems rarely go unrecognized today but lesser degrees of cardiac abnormality produced by hyper- or hypothyroid function are common and this factor may well result in the appreciation of a new dimension of thyrocardiac disorder.

ACTION OF THYROID HORMONES ON THE HEART

The active thyroid hormone is probably in the form of free circulating tri-iodothyronine (T3) which maintains a balance with its bound form, both being derived from the peripheral breakdown of the prohormone thyroxine (T4), itself circulating as a free and a protein bound moiety. A separate pathway of thyroxine metabolism also exists in that this substance may form either peripherally active T3 or an inactive compound reverse T3 (RT3). The true significance of RT3 is not understood but as it is produced in severe stress states, e.g. preterminal conditions and myocardial infarction, there is some reason to believe that it might be an inbuilt method of sparing surviving healthy cells of excessive or unwanted metabolic stress.[1] An interesting facet which may have a direct bearing on the role of reverse T3 is the mode of action of the anti-arrhythmic drug, amiodarone. This iodine-containing compound, apart from its property in prolonging the myocardial cell action potential, with impressive results in sino-atrial disease and in many other forms of arrhythmias, increases the level of circulating RT3.[2,3] Thyroid hormones exert a negative feedback effect on pituitary thyroid stimulating hormone, thyrotrophin (TSH), and there is almost certainly an additional negative feedback effect on thyroid releasing hormone (TRH) from the hypothalamus. Other pituitary and hypothalamic hormones are also involved; TRH stimulates prolactin secretion[4] and dopamine will inhibit TSH release in man.[5] The thyrotropin-producing cells of the anterior pituitary gland are very sensitive to changes in circulating thyroid hormone levels, even within the normal ranges of T4 and T3 and it may be that this factor is of prime importance in considering the endocrine regulation of cardiac performance both in health and disease. A discussion on the role of thyroid auto-immune factors is beyond the scope of this chapter but if a positive titre of antibodies is found in any cardiac disorder, this is an indication for the thorough application of thyroid function tests especially to detect any evidence of glandular hypofunction.

The circulatory change in thyroid disease is essentially one of a disturbance of supply and demand. The increased cellular activity in hyperthyroidism means increased blood supply and the heart responds hyperdynamically and hyperkinetically to accomplish this. But the burden is two-fold for the heart muscle itself forms part of the increased metabolic requirements; although speculative, this could be an important reason why the cardiac output is so disproportionately high even for the required metabolic increase. There is a direct effect on the heart by thyroid hormones, increasing chronotropism and inotropism of the cardiac muscle fibre, a maximal response which is well seen from the study of the systolic time intervals. The left ventricular contractile force is increased more than would be expected from a consideration of the Frank–Starling mechanism; the pre-ejection phase of the systolic time intervals decreases together with shortened or unaltered duration of electromechanical systole, i.e. the stroke volume augments as well as the heart rate.[6] Oxygen consumption is greatly increased and while the healthy heart can easily withstand this excessive response, this is not the case in the ageing or otherwise diseased organ. Arrhythmias occur, frequently with high output cardiac failure. Conversely, in hypothyroidism even the low cardiac output is sufficient to supply the minimal requirements of the hypothyroid metabolic state; but the hypothyroid heart is intolerant of any rapid increase in thyroxine replacement during the early stages of treatment, for it is incapable of coping with the increased circulatory and metabolic demand.

The action of thyroid hormones on the cardiac muscle cell is not fully understood and is undoubtedly complex. Experimentally there appears to be an increased rate of diastolic depolarization and a decreased duration of the action potential in sino-atrial node cells,[7,8] plainly relevant in considering the association of arrhythmias with thyroid disease. Activation of the cyclic AMP system is probably not an important factor in promoting the direct effects of thyroid hormone on the heart[9] but calcium mobility within the cell is likely to have an important role in increasing muscle contractility.[10] Morkin[11] has shown that there may well be altered properties of cardiac muscle contraction for he has produced good evidence that new myosin formation may occur in experimental hyperthyroidism. The role of catecholamines in hyperthyroidism remains controversial even though Buccino et al.[12] showed that, experimentally in the isolated cat papillary muscle preparation, the level of thyroid activity although profoundly affecting the intrinsic contractile state of cardiac muscle was independent of both noradrenaline stores and alterations in high energy phosphate. No increase in circulating catecholamines in hyperthyroidism has been shown to occur despite the clinical simulation of increased sympathetic discharge.[13] Williams and Lefkowitz[14] have described an increased number of beta-receptor binding sites on cardiac muscle cells in hyperthyroid rats and although this could equate with the impressive improvement obtained with propranolol clinically, it is equally known that propranolol will decrease the peripheral conversion of T4 to T3.[15] No single or precise answer to how thyroid hormones act on the heart is as yet apparent.

HYPOTHYROIDISM

A wide spectrum of clinical response to impaired thyroid function exists and, contrary to the hyperthyroid state where the accent is on excessive stimulation of the heart and circulatory system, metabolic inactivity results in cardiac hypofunction. Nevertheless, unless there is serious underlying separate cardiac disease, the heart will be able to cope with the requirements of the organism. No haemodynamic evidence of cardiac failure was disclosed in myxoedematous patients studied by Graettinger et al.[16] The ECG shows minor repolarization changes but occasionally gross T wave inversion occurs, highly suggestive at first sight of severe ischaemia but frequently this is not due to coronary disease as the abnormality reverts to normal with replacement therapy. Arrhythmias (usually recurrent ventricular tachycardia) have been reported[17–19] in the florid myxoedematous state and have even been successfully treated with thyroxine. The estimation of the serum creatinine phosphokinase in hypothyroidism, routinely requested because of the abnormal ECG, is a deceptive test for it may be much elevated; this is due to skeletal muscle metabolic changes and not related to the isoenzyme fraction from the heart.[20,21]

In myxoedema bradycardia is usually but not always evident, peripheral perfusion is poor with cold hands and subnormal temperature, the heart sounds are distant and the jugular venous pressure frequently raised. The latter is of interest for it is usually due to the slow heart rate, occasionally to pericardial effusion and rarely to cardiac failure. In fact, the presentation is one of restrictive heart muscle disease and provides an uncommon instance when the resolution of changes to normality may be easily followed over a short space of time. There is little data even now concerning histological and ultrastructural changes in the myocardium but not only is there evidence of muscle damage, albeit transient, and possibly effects of pericardial effusion, but infiltration with myxoedema material certainly occurs (*Figure 1*).

The cardiac silhouette radiologically is frequently increased simply due to the bradycardia but occasionally to pericardial effusion. Myxoedema of itself does not cause cardiac enlargement. Pericardial effusion is of academic interest in the majority of cases for it causes only diagnostic difficulty and is unusually of sufficient size to produce impairment in diastolic filling. Echocardiography is the only sure way of detecting the presence of fluid and is a positive test in about 30 per cent of patients with myxoedema, most of whom will have no clinical features of this condition.[22] With thyroxine replacement the fluid will rapidly disappear but occasionally the resolution is not synchronous with the return of the euthyroid state and the reason for this is obscure. Occasionally in unexplained bradycardia in an overtly well subject a routine serum thyroxine is found to be low and hypothyroidism proves to be the cause of the slow heart rate.

Anginal pain is infrequent in myxoedema but even when it occurs, possibly with a markedly abnormal ECG, it may disappear with thyroxine therapy. The latter circumstance raises the possibility that a reversible form of a hypertrophic-type cardiomyopathy may be present, as suggested by Santos et al.[23] but this study is based only on echocardiographic evidence. Nevertheless, angina can become a problem and although treated with thyroxine together with a beta-blocking drug it may be impossible to render the patient euthyroid because of worsening ischaemic pain. Under the circumstances underlying coronary disease is generally present but coronary angiography may be required to prove this for, as frequently occurs in euthyroid normal middle-aged females with chest pain, the coronary tree proves to be clear of disease. Treatment of the sub-thyroid state with thyroxine must always be cautious when coronary disease is present for the heart muscle is particularly sensitive to the increased metabolic drive. Left ventricular failure or severe angina with infarction may occur. Dosage of l-thyroxine should be no more than 0·025 mg for several weeks and thereafter only gradual increase, introducing propranolol should angina become a problem.

There are now reports of bypass surgery for coronary disease with myxoedema, operation being successful even before the patient is rendered euthyroid.[24] Coronary disease in the reported cases was severe but seems to have been more proximal (especially left main) than distal disease—an important factor which makes investigation of a patient with angina and myxoedema all the more worthwhile.

If coronary disease occurs in myxoedema then it would be equally expected to be present but to a lesser degree in minor forms of hypothyroidism and even in sub-thyroid states (premyxoedema). The association of a raised cholesterol level in patients who are euthyroid but who have positive thyroid antibodies has been described by Bastenie et al.[25] and Fowler and Swale[26] and it is claimed that recognition and treatment with thyroxine of this form of sub-clinical

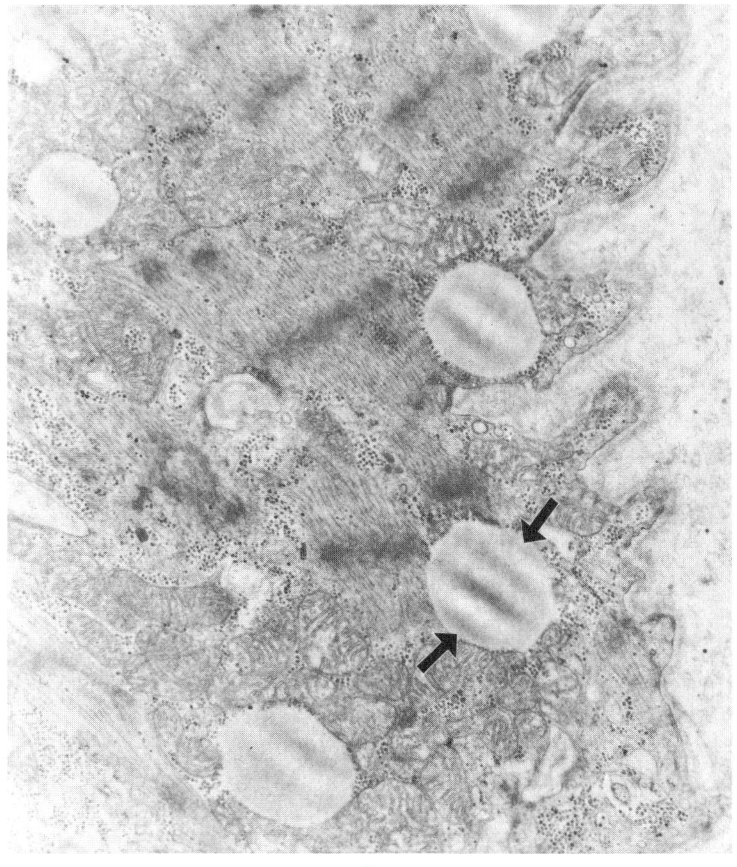

a

Figure 1. (a) Electron microscopy of muscle fibril from heart of a patient with severe coronary disease and myxoedema. Specimen taken during coronary by-pass procedure. The section (b) shows the presence of much glycogen, lipofuscin and numerous round masses of grey material, presumably myxoedema infiltration (arrow), in many areas totally replacing muscle fibril. (Courtesy of Mr. J. Parker and Professor M. J. Davies)

hypothyroidism may prevent progression to atherosclerotic disease.[27] On the other hand Tunbridge et al.,[28] in a wide survey of a normal population, could find no good evidence of association with coronary disease and auto-immune thyroid disorder. These findings are not supported by Tièche et al.,[29] whose study linked coronary artery disease with thyroid auto-immunity and raised TSH levels but not with hypercholesterolaemia. Despite a somewhat confused situation there is good rationale for Fowler's contention[27] and further work needs to be done. The effect of auto-immune disease in any of its forms on the heart

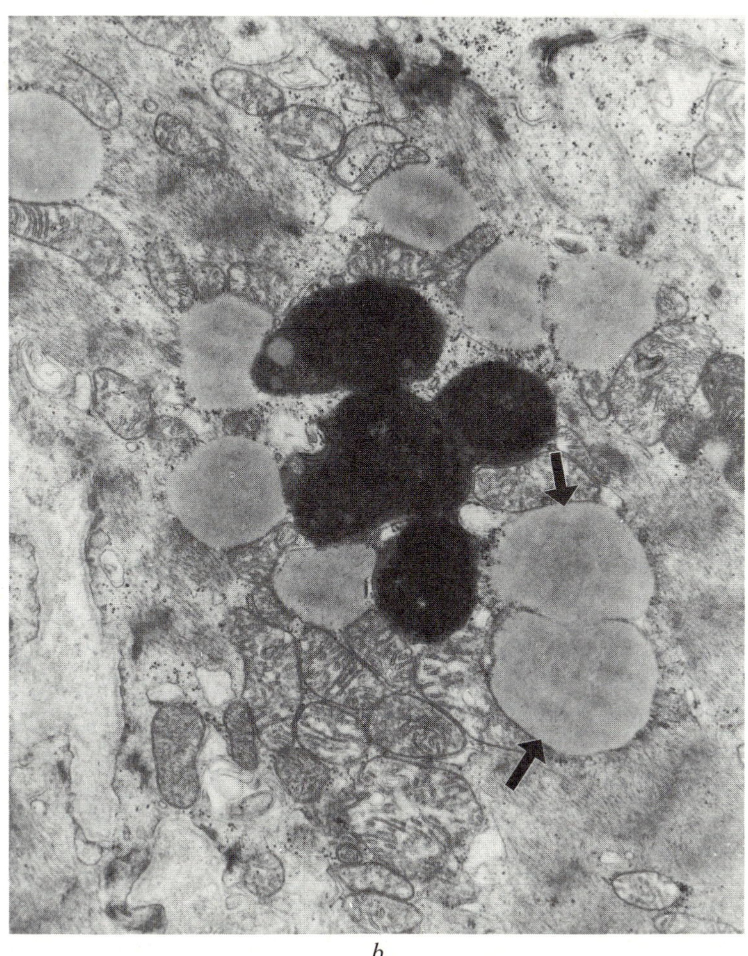

b

is unknown; as has been suggested by Matthews et al.[30] the auto-immune process itself may be invoked as a cause of vascular disease and the action on the cardiovascular system of circulating immune-complexes also needs to be explored. Symons and Colquhoun[31] looked at another aspect of symptomless auto-immune thyroid disease affecting the heart and have shown that rhythm disturbances frequently occur, postulating that abnormal depolarization and repolarization gradients occur in latent or absolute hypothyroidism and produce localized foci of instability, thus providing a basis for re-entry phenomena. The condition may mimic sino-atrial disease and it is conceivable that an auto-immune disorder will yet prove to have some bearing on the genesis of the sick-sinus syndrome.

HYPERTHYROIDISM

Heart disease in hyperthyroidism becomes of greater importance in the older patient. Classically in overt disease in the younger age groups hyperthyroidism generally gives rise to no cardiac problems at this time and changes in the cardiovascular system are overshadowed by the acute endocrine abnormality (*Figure 2a*). In later life the converse is true; usually the thyroid gland is not enlarged and eye signs are absent. Arrhythmias occur, especially paroxysmal or established atrial fibrillation, and it is only when thought is given to the nature of the possible high output circulatory state that hyperthyroidism is suspected. Other forms of arrhythmia are ventricular ectopics frequently in salvoes and multi-focal in character. Atrial flutter also occurs. Some indication of the difficulty in diagnosing hyperthyroidism as a cause of cardiac arrhythmia was given by a study of clinically euthyroid cardiac patients attending an out-patient department[32] and where it was found that 5 per cent of patients with proven permanent or paroxysmal atrial arrhythmias had underlying hyperthyroidism. An interesting and unexplained electrocardiographic abnormality occurring at any age is the prolonged PR interval, which returns to normal on regaining the euthyroid state.[33] Almost conversely, the Wolff–Parkinson–White syndrome has been reported and this abnormality disappears with euthyroidism.[34,35] Markedly inverted but transient T wave changes are commonly present in severe hyperthyroidism in younger patients and in the more acutely ill subject.

Of prime importance is the work by Forfar et al.,[36] who showed that in 75 consecutive patients with idiopathic atrial fibrillation a lack of response of TSH to TRH indicative of thyrotoxicosis was found in 10 (13 per cent of fibrillators), not all of whom had raised serum thyroid hormone levels. Eight reverted to stable sinus rhythm after treatment with ^{131}I or carbimazole, either spontaneously or after direct-current cardioversion. Covert thyrotoxicosis can therefore be identified consistently only by the failure of TSH levels to rise after TRH stimulation. Forfar et al.[37] have since described the successful reinstatement of sinus rhythm in patients with long-standing atrial fibrillation and a normal serum T4 and T3 but with failure of response of TSH to TRH, by a pre-treatment period with carbimazole.

Clinically the high output circulatory state explains most of the physical signs. Warm extremities are present from vasodilatation and increased blood flow, the pulse is full volume in character and the jugular venous pulsation easily seen. Biventricular enlargement is present, the first heart sound is loud, an apical third heart sound may be heard and a rough basal systolic bruit is audible in many cases. Ueda et al.[38] believe that the first heart sound is accentuated not because of tachycardia but by rapid closure of the mitral valve due to increased muscle contractility. It must be emphasized that the clinical presentation from the cardiac point of view may be insidious, and only the application of a routine thyroid function study in an otherwise idiopathic arrhythmia, or to elucidate the nature of some other form of cardiac disorder, will lead to the specific diagnosis of thyroid overactivity as a cause of the circulatory problem. Treatment of the thyroid state with carbimazole initially in all patients, and radio-iodine in a now ever decreasing number, will resolve the cardiac arrhythmia in the younger subject. Frequently in the older person the arrhythmia will remain and can only be satisfactorily treated by DC reversion (under anticoagulant cover), preferably as soon as the patient becomes euthyroid with treatment. Should the procedure be unsuccessful, these patients probably have specific heart muscle disease and require maintenance with digoxin and possibly diuretic therapy (*Figure 2b*). In hyperthyroidism the presence of cardiac failure, high-output congestive in type, is usually concomitant with rapid atrial fibrillation and is treated in the usual manner with digoxin, diuretics and of course carbimazole. A small dose of propranolol is frequently helpful in reducing the heart rate in the initial stages even in the presence of cardiac failure. Problems occasionally arise should some other cardiac condition be present, e.g. mitral or coronary artery disease or if the patient is pregnant.

HEART MUSCLE DISEASE

Hypertrophy of the heart muscle fibre is the experimental response to thyroid hormone[39–41] and there is reason to believe that a similar result occurs in man.[42] Now that sophisticated and non-invasive methods of assessing heart muscle thickness exist, e.g. the echocardiogram, there is good evidence of regression of cardiac hypertrophy from the hyperthyroid and even in hypothyroidism to the euthyroid stage.[42,43] It is known that during the acute stages of thyrotoxicosis, gross T wave changes may occur which rapidly become normal once the euthyroid status is regained. Cardiac dilatation as a response to long-standing thyroxine stimulation is more difficult to prove but undoubtedly in the older subject dilated heart muscle disease is encountered which does not regress when concomitant hyperthyroidism is fully treated. These cases are infrequent but nevertheless important for, combined with dysrhythmias, may be responsible for those patients with persistent unexplained cardiac failure. Additionally, cases where atrial fibrillation persists after the successful treatment of the hyperthyroid state and attempted DC reversion may be examples of specific heart muscle disease due to long-standing hyperthyroidism.

A fascinating myocardial response in a genetically susceptible subject is that of hypertrophic cardiomyopathy. Some evidence exists that thyroid hormone may be an important factor. This consideration is

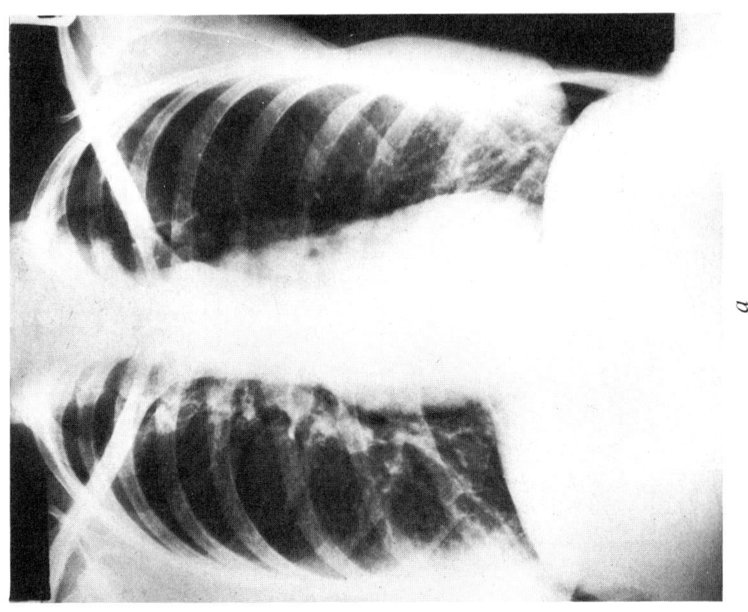

a

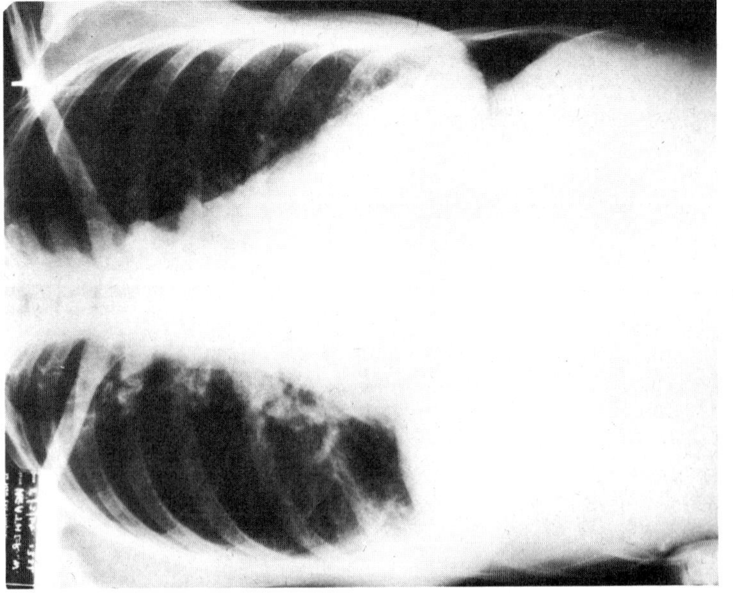

a

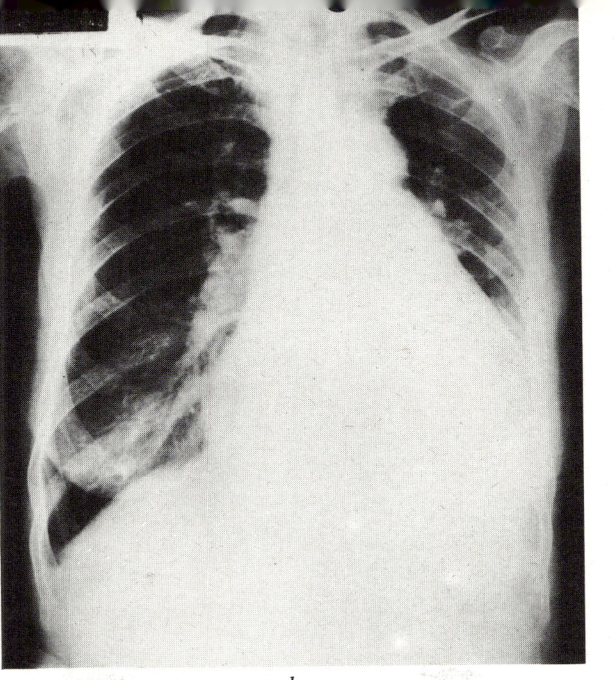

b

Figure 2. (a) Chest x-ray of female aged 40 years with hyperthyroidism and atrial fibrillation showing gross cardiac enlargement. The cardiac silhouette returns to normal size after successful anti-thyroid treatment and spontaneous reversion of sinus rhythm (film 1 year later). (b) Specific heart muscle disease in a patient aged 72 years who had hyperthyroidism, atrial fibrillation and congestive failure. Despite successful anti-thyroid treatment there was no alteration in heart size in the following 2 years.

based on the observation that thyroxine analogues were present in excess in the circulation of a patient with cardiac disease with considerable unexplained myocardial hypertrophy, and who later developed conventional hyperthyroidism.[44] With the knowledge that one of these analogues—viz. tri-iodothyroacetic acid (triac)—is a powerful stimulus of myocardial metabolism[41], a series of experiments were commenced to see if cardiac hypertrophy, either of ordinary type or even of hypertrophic variety, could be produced. Stimulus to this idea was provided by the disclosure that hypertrophic cardiomyopathy was found in several patients with thyrotoxicosis[45] and the relatively high incidence of hyperthyroidism in hypertrophic cardiomyopathy was later confirmed by Bell et al.[46] Subsequent experimental observations have shown that triac may cause myocardial cellular disarray similar to that seen in hypertrophic cardiomyopathy, but only if given early in life at a time when the heart muscle itself is actively growing.[47,48] These findings were obtained in the fetal heart of Wistar-strain rats but not in the heart of the pregnant mother to whom triac had been administered when pregnant. The relevance of these results to the association of hypertrophic cardiomyopathy and hyperthyroidism is as yet unclear but it suggests, from the consideration of the use of a number of other drugs used experimentally with triac to counteract hypertrophy, that it may be related to a disturbance of membrane stability arising at a vulnerable phase in heart muscle development, rather than some change in adreno-receptor status. This view fits with the fact that increased catecholamine levels have never been disclosed in hypertrophic disease either in the circulation or in the heart muscle cell, or in hyperthyroidism.

It has been suggested that much may be learnt of the response of the normal and diseased heart to the stimulus provided by thyroid hormones. In this context two patients with hypertrophic cardiomyopathy have been seen by the author who have entered a congestive phase, presumably a result of severe and untreated hyperthyroidism in the one and chronic overdosage with thyroid hormone in the other.

CONCLUSIONS

Few conditions in cardiovascular disease are as satisfying to treat as thyroid heart disorder. Ill health is transformed and the patient's overall improvement in well-being, whilst understandably attributed to a return to the euthyroid state, is frequently appreciated by the patient as a disappearance of troublesome ectopic beats, overactive heart or discomforting dyspnoea. For this result to occur early diagnosis is essential and the clinician must be aware of the wide spectrum of cardiovascular changes that may be produced in thyroid disease. Now that thyroid function studies are of such an order of sensitivity and selectivity, further abnormal cardiac conditions may well be disclosed attributable to thyroid abnormality. This remains to be seen.

REFERENCES

1. Chopra TJ, Chopra U, Smith SR, Reza M, Solomon DH. Reciprocal changes in serum concentrations of 3′3′5′ tri-iodothyronine (reverse T3) and 3′3′5 tri-iodothyronine (T3) in systemic illness. *J Clin Endocrinol Metab* 1975; **41**: 1043.
2. Burger A, Nicod P, Suter P, Vallotton MB, Vagenakis A, Braverman L. Reduced active thyroid hormone levels in acute illness. *Lancet* 1976; **1**: 653.
3. Jonckheer MH, Block P, Broeckaert I, Cornette C, Beckers C. ‘Low T3 syndrome’ in patients chronically treated with an iodine-containing drug, amiodarone. *Clin Endocrinol* 1978; **9**: 27.
4. Snyder PJ, Jacobs LS, Utiger RD, Danghaday WH. Thyroid hormone inhibition of the prolactin response to thyrotropin-releasing hormone. *J Clin Invest* 1973; **52**: 2324.
5. Besses GS, Burrow GN, Spaulding SW, Donabedian RK. Dopamine infusion acutely inhibits the TSH and prolactin response to TRH. *J Clin Endocrinol Metab* 1975; **41**: 985.
6. De Groot EJ, Leonard JJ. Hyperthyroidism as a high cardiac output state. *Am Heart J* 1970; **79**: 265.
7. Johnson PN, Freedberg AS, Marshall JM. Action of thyroid hormone on the transmembrane potential from sino-atrial cells and atrial muscle cells in isolated atria of rabbits. *Cardiology* 1973; **58**: 273.
8. Arnsdorf MF, Childers RW. Atrial electrophysiology in experimental hyperthyroidism in rabbits. *Circ Res* 1970; **26**: 575.
9. Levey GS, Skelton CL, Epstein SE. Influence of hyperthyroidism on the effects of norepinephrine on myocardial adenyl cyclase activity and contractile state. *Endocrinology* 1969; **85**: 1004.
10. Nayler WG, Merrilees NCR, Chipperfield D, Kurtz JB. Influence of hyperthyroidism on uptake and binding of calcium by cardiac microsomal fractions and on mitochondrial structure. *Cardiovasc Res* 1971; **5**: 469.
11. Morkin E. Stimulation of cardiac myosin adenosine triphosphatase in thyrotoxicosis. *Circ Res* 1979; **44**: 1.
12. Buccino RA, Spann JF Jr, Pool PE, Sonnenblick EH, Braunwald E. Influence of the thyroid state on the intrinsic contractile properties and energy stores of the myocardium. *J Clin Invest* 1967; **46**: 1669.
13. Coulombe P, Dussault JH, Walker P. Plasma catecholamine concentrations in hyperthyroidism and hypothyroidism. *Metabolism.* 1976; **25**: 973.
14. Williams LT, Lefkowitz RJ. Thyroid hormone regulation of β-adrenergic receptor number. *J Biol Chem* 1977; **252**: 2787.
15. Kallner G, Ljunggren JC, Tryselius M. The effect of propranolol on serum levels of T4, T3 and reverse T3 in hyperthyroidism. *Acta Med Scand* 1978; **204**: 35.
16. Graettinger JS, Muenster JJ, Checchia CS, Grissom RL, Campbell JA. Correlation of clinical and haemodynamic studies of patients with hypothyroidism. *J Clin Invest* 1958; **37**: 502.
17. Ohler WR, Abramson J. The heart in myxoedema. *Arch Intern Med* 1934; **53**: 165.
18. Hansen JE. Paroxysmal ventricular tachycardia associated with myxoedema. A case report. *Am Heart J* 1961; **61**: 692.
19. Lim CH, Lim P. Recurrent ventricular tachycardia in hypothyroidism. *Aust NZ J Med* 1976; **6**: 68.

20. Graig FA, Ross G. Serum creatine-phosphokinase in thyroid disease. *Metabolism* 1963; **12**: 57.
21. Doran GR, Wilkinson JH. The origin of the elevated activities of creatine kinase and other enzymes in the sera of patients with myxoedema. *Clin Chim Acta* 1975; **62**: 203.
22. Kerber RE, Sherman B. Echocardiographic evaluation of pericardial effusion in myxoedema. *Circulation* 1975; **52**: 823.
23. Santos AD, Miller RP, Mathew PK, Wallace WA, Cave WT Jr, Hinojosa L. Echocardiographic characterization of the reversible cardiomyopathy of hypothyroidism. *Am J Med* 1980; **68**: 675.
24. Paine TD, Rogers WJ, Baxley WA, Russell RO. Coronary arterial surgery in patients with incapacitating angina pectoris and myxoedema. *Am J Cardiol* 1977; **40**: 226.
25. Bastenie PA, Bonnyns M, Neve P, Van Haelst L, Chailly M. Clinical and pathological significance of symptomatic and atrophic thyroiditis. *Lancet* 1967; **1**: 915.
26. Fowler PBS, Swale J. Premyxoedema and coronary disease. *Lancet* 1967; **1**: 1077.
27. Fowler PBS, Swale J. Andrews H. Hypercholesterolaemia in borderline hypothyroidism. *Lancet* 1970; **2**: 488.
28. Tunbridge WMG, Evered DC, Hall R et al. The spectrum of thyroid disease in a community: the Whickham Survey. *Clin Endocrinol* 1977; **7**: 481.
29. Tièche M, Lupi AG, Gutzwiller F, Grob PJ, Studer H, Bürgi H. Borderline low thyroid function and thyroid autoimmunity: risk factors for coronary heart disease. *Br Heart J* 1981; **46**: 202.
30. Mathews JD, Whittingham S, Mackay JR. Auto-immune mechanisms in human vascular disease. *Lancet* 1974; **2**: 1423.
31. Symons C, Colquhoun MC. Asymptomatic thyroiditis and atrial dysrhythmias. *Proceedings of the XVth International Congress of Therapeutics, Brussels, September 1979*. Amsterdam: Excerpta Medica, 1980: Theme I: 137–43.
32. Symons C, Myers A, Kingstone D, Boss M. Response to thyrotrophin-releasing hormone in atrial dysrhythmias. *Postgrad Med J* 1978; **54**: 658.
33. Hoffman I, Lowrey RD. The electrocardiogram and thyrotoxicosis. *Am J Cardiol* 1960; **6**: 893.
34. Strong JA. Thyrotoxicosis with ophthalmoplegia, myopathy, Wolff–Parkinson–White syndrome and pericardial friction. *Lancet* 1949; **1**: 959.
35. Sanghvi LM, Banerjee K. Wolff–Parkinson–White syndrome associated with thyrotoxicosis. *Am J Cardiol* 1961; **8**: 431.
36. Forfar JC, Miller HC, Toft AD. Occult thyrotoxicosis: a correctable cause of 'idiopathic' atrial fibrillation. *Am J Cardiol* 1979; **44**: 9.
37. Forfar JC, Feek CM, Miller HC, Toft AD. Atrial fibrillation and isolated suppression of the pituitary-thyroid axis: response to antithyroid therapy. *Int J Cardiol* 1981; **1**: 43.
38. Ueda H, Uozumi Z, Watanabe H et al. Phonocardiographic study of hyperthyroidism. *Japan. Heart J* 1963; **4**: 509.
39. Sandler G, Wilson GM. The production of cardiac hypertrophy by thyroxine in the rat. *Q J Exp Physiol* 1959; **44**: 282.
40. Cohen J, Aroesty JM, Rosenfeld MG. Determinants of thyroxine induced cardiac hypertrophy in mice. *Circ Res* 1966; **18**: 388.
41. Symons C, Olsen EGJ, Hawkey CM. The production of cardiac hypertrophy by tri-iodothyroacetic acid. *J Endocrinol* 1975; **65**: 341.
42. Sandler G, Wilson GM. The nature and prognosis of heart disease in thyrotoxicosis. *Q J Med* 1959; **28**: 347.
43. Nixon JV, Anderson RJ, Cohen ML. Alterations in left ventricular mass and performance in patients treated effectively for thyrotoxicosis: a comparative echocardiographic study. *Am J Med* 1979; **67**: 268.
44. Symons C, Richardson PJ, Wood JB. Unusual presentation of thyrocardiac disease. *Lancet* 1971; **2**: 1163.

45. Symons C, Richardson PJ, Feizi O. Hypertrophic cardiomyopathy and hyperthyroidism: a report of 3 cases. *Thorax* 1974; **29**: 713.
46. Bell R, Barber PV, Bray CL, Beton DC. Incidence of thyroid disease in cases of hypertrophic cardiomyopathy. *Br Heart J* 1978; **40**: 1306.
47. Olsen EGJ, Symons C, Hawkey CM. Effect of triac on the developing heart. *Lancet* 1977; **2**: 221.
48. Hawkey CM, Olsen EGJ, Symons C. Production of cardiac muscle abnormalities in offspring of rats receiving tri-iodothyroacetic acid (triac) and the effect of beta adrenergic blockade. *Cardiovasc Res* 1981; **15**: 196.

Chapter 8

Sarcoid heart disease

Hugh A. Fleming

INTRODUCTION

Sarcoid heart disease was generally considered to be a rare condition but, as will be demonstrated in this chapter, it occurs more commonly than is clinically recognized. Scadding[1] defined sarcoid as a 'disease characterised by the presence in all of several affected organs or tissues of epithelial cell tubercles without caseation'. He stated that the organs most frequently involved were the lymph nodes, lung, liver, spleen, skin, eyes, small bones of the hands and feet and the salivary glands, although every organ and tissue, with the possible exception of the adrenals, was reported to have been involved. It is of interest that no specific mention was given to the heart in this list.

In 1929, the first patient with sarcoid heart disease was described by Bernstein et al.[2] and, in 1937, Gentzen[3] reported the first death from sarcoid heart disease. Thereafter, there were many case reports, particularly in Negroes from the southern states of the U.S.A.,[4] and these may well have been responsible for the widely accepted, but unproved, view that this race was particularly susceptible to sarcoid heart disease.

In the United Kingdom the first case of sarcoid heart disease was described by Forbes and Usher[5] in 1962: a 44-year-old steel worker who died from heart disease. There was massive involvement of the left ventricle by sarcoidosis and, typically, minimal disease of other organs. As a result of six reported necropsy cases[6] it was evident that sarcoid heart disease was a much more frequently encountered condition than had hitherto been realized, and the author's national survey was commenced. This was by its nature limited but by 1974 50 cases were reported, 20 of them with necropsy confirmation.[7]

In 1976 the Japanese reported 42 necropsy cases[8] and in 1977 a large American series[9] analysed current information extensively although they omitted to include the Japanese and British series—probably the reason why stress was given to the Negro as being particularly susceptible to sarcoid heart disease, something which has not been borne out by the reports from either Japan or Great Britain.

SARCOID HEART DISEASE: THE BRITISH STUDY

The collection of cases of patients with sarcoid heart disease began in 1971, is continuing, and this chapter describes this experience. Strict criteria are applied for inclusion in this series. The prime requirement is that there must be a cardiac condition which is compatible with sarcoid. This really amounts to any bizarre form of heart disease for which there is no other aetiological explanation. Next, there must be a clinical diagnosis of sarcoidosis as a multi-system disease, and wherever possible there should be histological evidence of the pathological process that is sarcoidosis. The only certain category is necropsy confirmation. Cases where the diagnosis is not sufficiently certain are not included in the series but are followed up for their interest. Patients studied are restricted to those from the United Kingdom. To date there are 163 cases, 87 males and 76 females.

Distribution of Patients

Although the diagnosis of sarcoid heart disease is not made as frequently as the true incidence of the disease warrants, this does not entirely explain the interesting distribution of cases. Of 163 patients, 62 come from East Anglia. East Anglia has a population of under 2 000 000 people and there is no reason to suspect that sarcoidosis of itself has a high incidence in that part of the country, although a more detailed investigation is planned to look into this, as this contrasts with the very few patients who have been reported from the northern part of the United Kingdom.

Cardiac Presentation

In this study the vast majority of the patients presented with cardiac symptoms and signs: 47 of 163 patients died suddenly and in 26 of them death was the presentation. Complete heart block occurred in 33, a congestive-type specific heart muscle disease in 27, and various forms of arrhythmia (extrasystoles and both supraventricular and ventricular tachycardia) and resistance to treatment were very common. Partial heart block and bundle branch block, especially right, were also encountered. A myocardial infarction-like presentation occurred in some patients and there were a few with pericarditis. Haemodynamically significant valve involvement was uncommon. Mitral systolic murmurs, which may be transient, were frequently heard, presumably due to papillary muscle dysfunction. In only two cases has papillary muscle damage been such that mitral valve replacement has been necessary.

Illustrative Case Histories

Apart from instances of sudden death, many of the histories are long and involved, and obviously confusing to the attending physician. The first case[4, 5] illustrates many of the typical features of the disease and also the difficulty of defining prognosis and the value of treatment. This was a female not diagnosed in life. At necropsy at the age of 59 years her left ventricle was extensively infiltrated with fibrogranulomatous lesions typical of sarcoidosis. Her hospital file contained electrocardiograms recorded over a period of 8 years.[7] In 1961 a tachycardia with left bundle branch block occurred; 2 days after this sinus rhythm was present still with left bundle branch block. Six years later she was in complete heart block; the following year there were multifocal ventricular premature systoles and a month later she was in sinus rhythm with normal QRS complexes and only slight prolongation of the PR interval. This was the best electrocardiogram that she had ever had and was in fact very nearly normal. This satisfactory electrocardiographic progress could have been regarded as a favourable sign either of spontaneous improvement or the result of any particular treatment given; yet she died suddenly a few days later and the necropsy demonstrated her heart was extensively involved with active sarcoidosis.

Another previously documented case was a 34-year-old man who was found dead on a motorway. At necropsy the pathologist found that apart from the trauma, all the organs were macroscopically normal but on routine histological examination sarcoid granulomata were scattered throughout the usual organs and in particular in the myocardium and the ventricular septum. *Figure 1* shows a typical granuloma under the epicardium of the left ventricle. It is of interest that three of the patients in this series have been involved in road traffic accidents although the circumstances were too ill-defined for any profitable conclusions to be made. However, this raises the possibility that sarcoid heart disease in airline pilots may have to be considered in the context of air-safety control.

The third case was a problem of complete heart block in a 60-year-old man who was paced satisfactorily until he died from pacemaker failure. His heart weighed 890 g and was infiltrated by numerous large white fleshy nodules, particularly in the left ventricular wall and ventricular septum (*Figure 2*). This looked to the pathologist like a

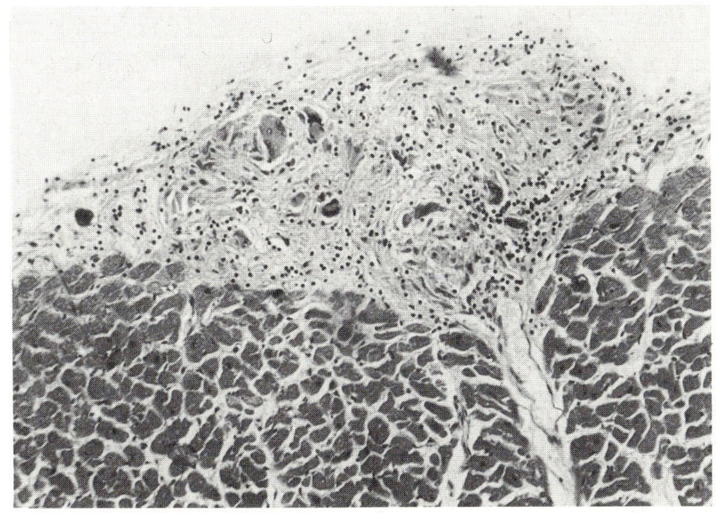

Figure 1. Sarcoid granuloma under the pericardium over the left ventricle of a 34-year-old man who died suddenly. The heart and other organs were macroscopically normal.

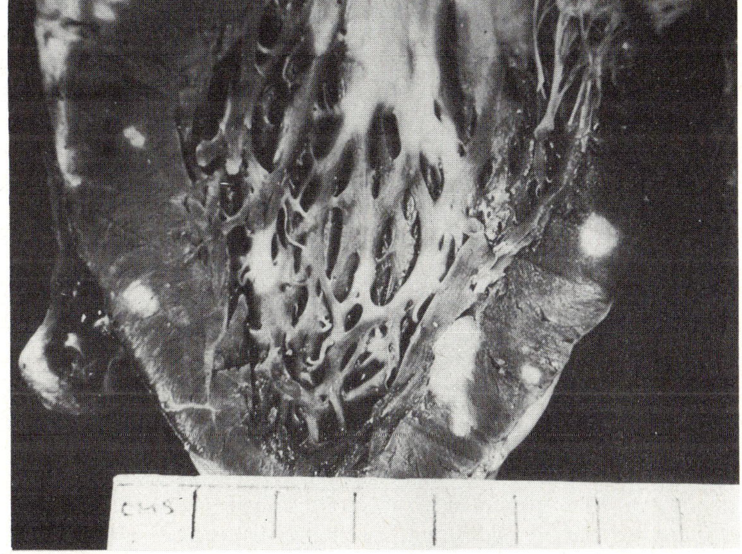

Figure 2. The left ventricle and ventricular septum of a 60-year-old man who died with heart block. The white masses in the left ventricular wall and occupying the septum macroscopically resemble tumour.

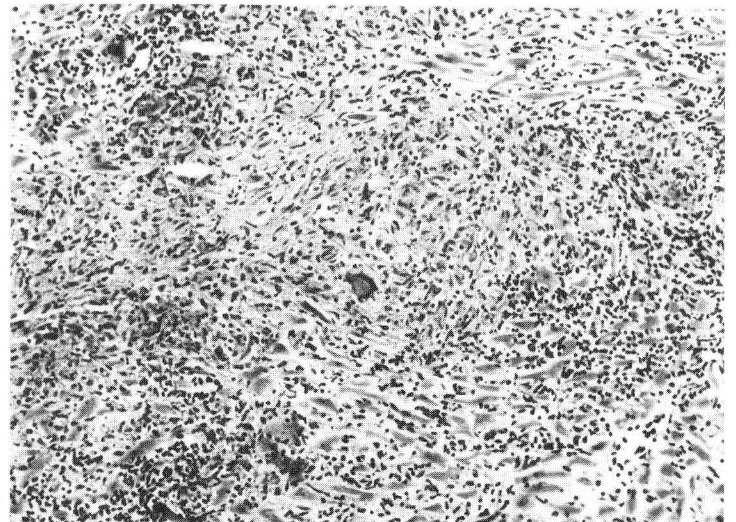

Figure 3. Microscopy of the left ventricle. Giant cell granulomata largely replacing myocardial fibres, the residue of which can still be seen.

tumour until microscopy showed the sarcoid granulomata. The findings have been reported in detail elsewhere.[10]

Patient 4 demonstrates how the heart can be massively involved and yet the subject led a relatively normal life until the terminal event. This 30-year-old man was playing football when he collapsed and was admitted to hospital with a very fast tachycardia which was difficult to control. The electrocardiogram was consistent with transmural myocardial infarction, bundle branch block and varying degrees of AV dissociation (but without bradycardia). He was eventually able to return to work but died suddenly and at necropsy his heart weighed 850 g, much of this being due to confluent active sarcoid granulomata. In this instance, as in a number of others, it was surprising that the cardiac condition was compatible with life at all, much less a normal and physically active life. As in other similar cases, the sarcoid involvement of other organs was inconspicuous but microscopically there was extensive involvement of lymph nodes, lung, liver and spleen, emphasizing this is a generalized systemic disease and not a localized heart disorder, as may be seen in giant cell myocarditis.

An example of one of the few black people in this series was a young West Indian who presented with severe congestive cardiac failure, mitral regurgitation and intractable rhythm problems. He also had clinical evidence of eye and mediastinal sarcoidosis and the Kveim test was positive. The diagnosis of sarcoid heart disease was made in life and he was treated energetically, including steroid therapy, but died in

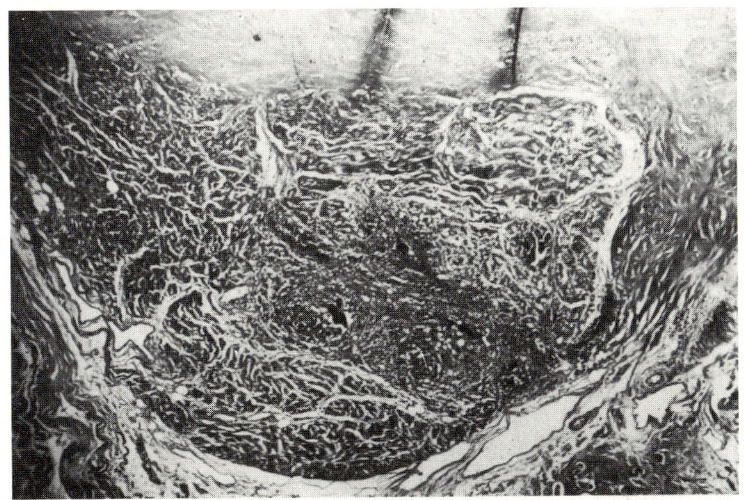

Figure 4. Conducting system. Granulomata with giant cells entirely replace the main bundle of His, and also its right and left branches.

congestive heart failure. At necropsy the heart was extensively involved (*Figure 3*) with replacement of the papillary muscles of the mitral valve. Detailed studies of the conducting system showed that the right bundle in particular was entirely replaced by the granulomatous process (*Figure 4*). It is not surprising, therefore, that rhythm problems, and, in particular, heart block are common in this condition.

A further patient presented with a hypertrophic cardiomyopathy-type syndrome.[11] This was due to massive involvement of the ventricular septum with sarcoid granulomata which encroached on the left ventricular outflow tract and it was only at necropsy that the true diagnosis was made.

The last case illustrates some of the difficulties of prognosis and assessment of treatment—a woman aged 35, unusual in this series in that she presented with pulmonary sarcoidosis. At the age of 31 her first electrocardiogram showed complete heart block. Due to a severe Cushingoid reaction from previous steroid treatment, the patient refused further medical treatment and also permanent pacing. She has since been followed up, sinus rhythm has returned, and there has been frequent ambulant ECG monitoring. During this time no active treatment has been given and from 1978 to date the only ECG abnormality has been a slightly prolonged PR interval with normal ventricular complexes. Twenty-four hour ECG tapes have been satisfactory. It is hoped that her prognosis is good, but remembering the first case described above who eventually died, also with a near-normal electrocardiogram, the prognosis must remain guarded.

Evidence of Sarcoid in Other Organs

The diagnosis of sarcoidosis is dependent on the presence of multi-system disease and ultimately is a histological diagnosis. In this series of 163 patients the following biopsies were positive:

Kveim test	66	(21 others negative)	Lung	5
Lymph nodes	23		Eye	1
Skin	11		Bone	1
Liver	10		Heart	1

We now feel that transbronchial pulmonary biopsy may be a satisfactory way of obtaining histological evidence. Where positive, the Kveim test is useful but negatives can be misleading. We have examples of negative Kveim in necropsy proven cases. Endomyocardial biopsy is plainly valuable when positive but because of the patchy distribution of the disease a negative result is of limited value. One patient has had mitral valve replacement and at surgery the gross diagnosis of sarcoid heart disease was confirmed. The excised papillary muscles had been entirely replaced by sarcoid granulomatous tissue and yet both the Kveim and endomyocardial biopsy have subsequently been repeatedly negative.

ECG Appearances

ECG analysis has been possible in most of the cases and the following abnormalities were noted:

Bundle-branch block (especially right)	60
Ventricular ectopic beats	46
Ventricular tachycardia	21
Complete heart block	34
Supraventricular tachycardia	40
Partial heart block	29
T wave changes	37
Myocardial infarction	10
Total	277

The total figure is due to the fact that any one case may appear under more than one heading.

Organ Involvement in 163 Cases Other than the Heart

Lung	65	Liver	10
Lymph nodes	34	Nerves	8
Skin	33	Bone	5
Eye	31	Parotid	5
Spleen	11		

It is also seen infrequently in the uterus, pituitary, meninges, kidney and thyroid.

FURTHER INVESTIGATION

This collection of cases was started chiefly to evaluate the frequency of occurrence of sarcoid heart disease. The study is continuing by annual review in the hope that useful therapeutic and prognostic information will emerge. The most rewarding tests appear to be ambulant monitoring and also echocardiography, studying particularly the left ventricular wall motion and the mitral valve. Radioisotope scanning may be useful in demonstrating lesions larger than one centimetre and angiotensin-converting enzyme estimations may be of assistance in assessing sarcoid activity and in helping to decide how energetic treatment should be.

TREATMENT

Obviously any arrhythmia, heart block, or heart failure must be treated on its own merits. Pacing is obligatory in heart block and every known cardiac drug has been used in the difficult arrhythmias. The difficulty is to decide if, and when, to use steroids and how useful they will be. In isolated case reports benefit has been reported in some patients but, as previously emphasized, the spontaneous variations in the natural history of the disease makes such observations impossible to evaluate.

Table 1
Table of deaths

	70	(of 163 cases in series)
Necropsy in	53	
Male	32	Age range 19–74 (mean 45·7)
Female	21	Age range 26–77 (mean 48·8)
	22	In East Anglia—3 in Ely
Sudden deaths	45	
	26	Not previously diagnosed
Black patients	5	

However the figures shown in Table 1 regarding deaths are so impressive that if there is doubt about whether or not to embark on steroid therapy these should be prescribed as the prognosis is otherwise so poor.

CONCLUSIONS

Several points have emerged from the present and other surveys:

1. Sarcoid heart is not rare.
2. It is often not part of the florid picture of general sarcoidosis.
3. The heart may be massively involved when other organs are only minimally affected.

4. Any part of the heart may be involved but the muscular ventricular septum is most commonly infiltrated and detailed histological study is required.
5. Cardiac presentation can take any form and sarcoid heart disease should be strongly considered in any bizarre form of cardiac disease for which there is no other explanation.
6. Sarcoid heart disease should particularly be suspected where there are difficult and varied disorders of rhythm.
7. Sudden death is common and may be the mode of presentation.

Finally, the diagnosis of sarcoid heart disease will only be made if there is a high index of suspicion, and if histological confirmation of the condition is diligently sought.

It should be noted that this study is continuing and the total number of patients now exceeds 250.

ACKNOWLEDGMENTS

I am indebted to numerous colleagues and their secretaries for their help and in particular to Mrs. Sheila Bailey who has collated the great amount of material that has been collected. Thanks are also due to Mrs. Anita Mead for secretarial assistance, and to Dr. P. G. I. Stovin for pathological advice.

REFERENCES

1. Scadding JG. *Sarcoidosis*. London: Eyre & Spottiswoode, 1967: 291.
2. Bernstein M, Konzleman FW, Sidlick DM. Boeck's sarcoid. (Report of a case with visceral involvement.) *Arch Intern Med* 1929; **44**: 721.
3. Gentzen G. Über Riesenzellen granulome bei zwei Fällen von Endocardfibrose. *Beitr Pathol* 1937; **98**: 375.
4. Lorell B, Alderman EL, Mason JW. Cardiac sarcoidosis. Diagnosis with endomyocardial biopsy and treatment with corticosteroids. *Am J Cardiol* 1978; **42**: 143.
5. Forbes G, Usher A. Fatal myocardial sarcoidosis. *Br Med J* 1962; **2**: 771.
6. Ghosh P, Fleming HA, Gresham GA, Stovin PGI. Myocardial sarcoidosis. *Br Heart J* 1972; **34**: 769.
7. Fleming HA. Sarcoid heart disease. *Br Heart J* 1974; **35**: 54.
8. Matsui Y, Iwai K, Tachibana T et al. Clinicopathological study of fatal myocardial sarcoidosis. *Ann NY Acad Sci* 1976; **278**: 455.
9. Roberts WC, McAllister HA, Ferrans VJ. Sarcoidosis of the heart. A clinicopathologic study of 35 necropsy patients (group I) and review of 78 previously described necropsy patients (group II). *Am J Med* 1977; **63**: 86.
10. Fawcett FJ, Goldberg MJ. Heart block resulting from myocardial sarcoidosis. *Br Heart J* 1974; **36**: 220.
11. Awdeh MR, Erwin S, Young JM, Nunn S. Systolic anterior motion of the mitral valve caused by sarcoid involving the septum. *South Med J* 1978; **2**: 1146.

Chapter 9

Alcohol-induced heart muscle disease

Peter J. Richardson and Alex A. Wodak

INTRODUCTION

Ethyl alcohol is a volatile liquid produced by the action of yeast upon organic matter. This process of fermentation has been known for over 5000 years and is widespread among all cultures apart from the Muslim world.

The process of fermentation of alcohol produces other volatile compounds known as 'congeners' which contribute to the taste of individual types of alcohol. However, almost the entire range of damaging effects is attributed to ethyl alcohol itself or to its breakdown products. There is no evidence that the type of alcohol influences the type or the extent of the complications. Damage appears to be more common with consistent heavy drinking rather than sporadic binge drinking. Liver damage from alcohol is closely correlated with average daily consumption and duration of drinking. There is a vast overlap, however, with some individuals developing complications before others. In addition there is, at present, no adequate explanation for the pattern of 'target organ' damage, whereby some individuals who abuse alcohol develop problems in one organ system rather than another. At present the relationship of alcohol consumption to disease has been most closely studied in liver disease and this knowledge extrapolated to other organs. It is possible in certain circumstances that other systems will prove to be more susceptible to damage from alcohol.

Since World War II, a spectacular increase in consumption of alcohol has taken place throughout the Western world. In Britain, the annual per capita consumption of alcohol has almost doubled in 30 years to exceed 7 litres of absolute alcohol. *Figure 1* shows consumption of beer, wines and spirits in the UK 1960–80 using 1970 as a

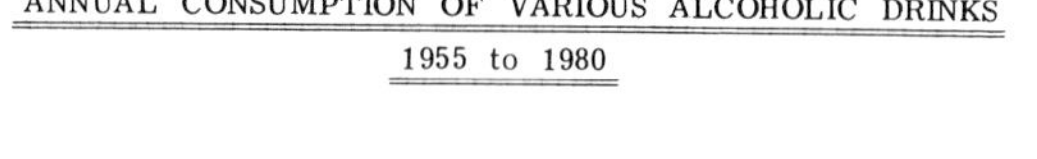

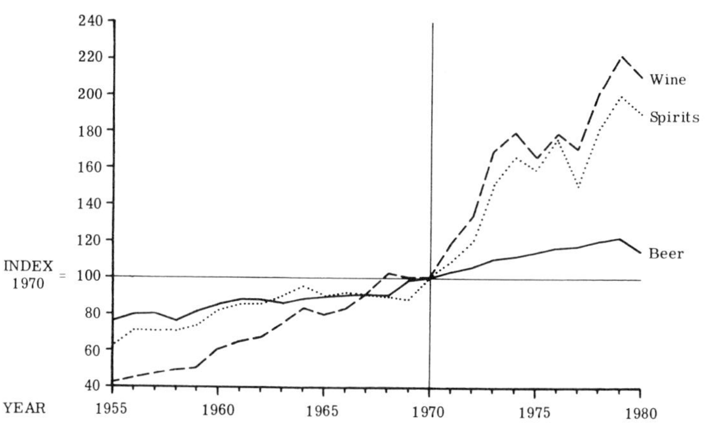

Figure 1. Consumption of beer, wines and spirits from 1955 to 1980 calculated from official excise figures. (Reproduced by kind permission of Dr. J.B. Saunders.)

base year. This demonstrates a slight rise in consumption during 1960–70 which accelerated during 1970–80. *Figure 2* sets out the annual per capita consumption of alcohol and cirrhosis mortality in Western countries in the late 1970s, showing a close correlation between these.[1] The use of cirrhosis mortality figures in the epidemiology of alcohol-related diseases is firmly established as the post mortem changes are well defined and the non-alcohol causes of cirrhosis scarcely fluctuate. Unfortunately there is no equivalent 'gold standard' for the study of the epidemiology of alcoholic heart disease.

In England, as in most other Western countries, increases have been noted in all statistics of alcohol-related problems and it is likely that heart disease related to alcohol abuse has also increased. Apart from the recent overall increase in drinking, there is particular concern that the current high consumption pattern now affecting young people may result in a steady increase in alcohol-related diseases as this cohort ages.

In its 1979 report,[2] the Royal College of Psychiatrists recommended a safe limit of eight units a day for men and six units a day for women (a unit being the equivalent of half a pint of beer, a single of spirits, a glass of table wine or a glass of fortified wine, and approximating to 10 g of absolute alcohol). By contrast, Pequignot et al,[3] in a survey of drinking habits of 381 cirrhotics compared to a control population, detected a significantly increased risk of developing cirrhosis at the lower dose of 60 g a day for men and 20–40 g a day for women. Threshold levels of

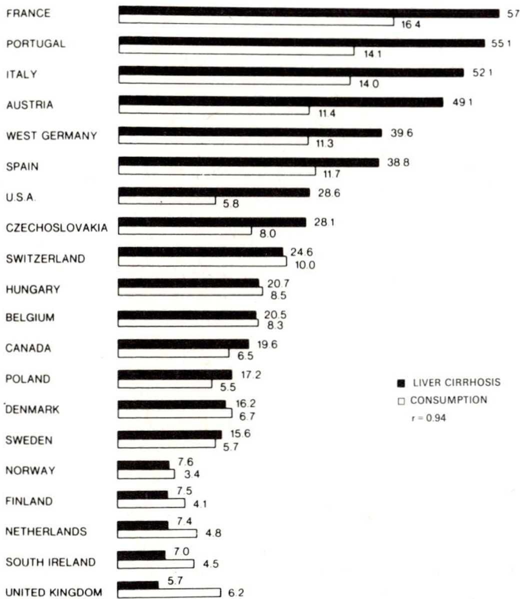

Figure 2. Correlation between mortality from alcoholic cirrhosis per 100 000 population and alcohol consumption per capita (litres) in Western countries.

alcohol consumption in relation to myocardial damage have not been quantitated. Table 1 sets out alcohol content of commonly consumed alcoholic beverages.

Table 1
Alcohol content of alcoholic beverages

Beverage	*Quantity*	*Alcohol content* (g)	*Alcohol strength* (% v/v)
Beer	Pint	16	2–4
Fortified wine (e.g. sherry)	Bottle	110	18–20
Table wine	Bottle (70 cl)	70	10–12
Spirit	Bottle (26 oz.)	240	40

1. Figures refer to alcoholic beverages on sale in the United Kingdom.
2. Ten grams of alcohol contained in (approximately):
   $\frac{1}{2}$ pint of beer
   1 glass of sherry
   1 glass of wine
   1 single of spirit.

POPULATION AT RISK

A recent survey of drinking patterns in adults in England and Wales estimated that, overall, 6 per cent of men and 1 per cent of women exceed the specified safe limits.[4] Higher proportions of heavy drinkers were found in subsections of the population, notably the young (18–24 years), single (divorced/separated), unemployed men, working women with no children and certain occupations (construction, drinks industry). The Office of Health Economics estimates that during the 1970s in England and Wales there were 3 million heavy drinkers, 700 000 problem drinkers and 150 000 alcohol dependent. In the United States a recent report to Congress estimated 10 million adults and 3·3 million youths are problem drinkers.

DEFINITION

The definition of the cardiomyopathies has been revised by Goodwin and Oakley[5] and subsequently by the Cardiomyopathy Task Force.[6] The term cardiomyopathy should now be reserved for heart muscle disease of unknown cause and association. The term specific heart muscle disease is used where the aetiological agent is known. Alcoholic cardiomyopathy should now accordingly be redefined as Alcoholic Heart Muscle Disease (AHMD). This is diagnosed when heart failure (cardiomegaly, dilated left ventricle and poor contractile function) in an alcohol abuser cannot be attributed to coronary arterial disease, valvar heart disease, hypertension or other specific cause. It should be remembered that alcohol may have a variety of effects on the heart which include arrhythmias, hypertension, the effects of congeners and contaminants, as well as nutritional deficiencies and this might be a cause of cardiac symptoms even when the heart muscle is not affected.

Amongst patients consuming large amounts of alcohol, it has been recognized that heart failure may be due not only to the direct effect of alcohol but also to a nutritional deficiency, particularly thiamine.[7] This condition usually presents as a high-output form and is well described (Shoshin beri-beri).[8,9] Similarly, the specific heart muscle disease due to cobalt is no longer seen.[10]

RELATION BETWEEN ALCOHOL CONSUMPTION AND MYOCARDIAL DISEASE

Although there is little doubt that alcohol abuse is associated with an increased risk of AHMD, there is no recent information on how much alcohol can be safely drunk without risk of myocardial damage. For any given exposure to alcohol, there is a wide spectrum of myocardial injury and undoubtedly the response is modified by pre-existing cardiac disease and individual susceptibility.

The association of alcohol abuse with arrhythmias and hypertension is well established though not frequently emphasized. The earliest recognition of an association between alcohol abuse and hypertension was made in 1915,[11] then neglected for 60 years until renewed interest prompted several important papers[12,13,13a] and a comprehensive review.[14] It is now well established that the risk of hypertension increases with alcohol consumption. Following abstinence the blood pressure usually returns to normal. Further work will be needed to establish the threshold level of consumption likely to result in hypertension and also to determine the factors that predispose to the development of an elevated blood pressure. The contribution made by hypertension to the excess mortality in heavy drinkers is also unknown.

Although most attention has focused on the complications of excessive alcohol consumption, in recent years evidence has accumulated that moderate drinkers have a lower cardiovascular mortality than abstainers or heavy drinkers.[15,16] Several well-designed studies, in addition to global comparisons of per capita consumption and deaths from myocardial infarction, have supported these conclusions. The upper and lower limits of alcohol consumption beyond which cardiovascular mortality begins to increase remain poorly defined.[17]

EPIDEMIOLOGY

The exact incidence of AHMD is not known because of a general reluctance to assess alcohol consumption and the difficulties in establishing a precise diagnosis. However, an indication of the importance of alcohol abuse in heart disease can be gained from the following.

Mortality Studies in Heavy Drinkers

Schmidt and Popham[18] reported 9889 males from Ontario, Canada, with a confirmed mean alcohol consumption nine times greater than a control population. The study involved 85 641 person years of observation during which 1823 deaths were recorded: 575 deaths from atherosclerotic and degenerative heart disease were observed (400 expected) ($p < 0{\cdot}01$) and this represented the largest group of deaths (32 per cent). In the same study liver disease accounted for 157 deaths (9 per cent). The association of the excess of observed deaths remained significant even after correcting for cigarette smoking.

Post-mortem Studies

Schenk and Cohen[19] reviewed 2100 consecutive post mortems in which 97 (4·5 per cent) of the patients drank to excess. Of these 97 patients, 21 per cent had clinical heart failure. The heart weight exceeded 300 g in all but 7 patients and 27 patients had heart weights over 500 g. Morgan[20] reported a post mortem study of 240 patients dying of alcoholic cirrhosis. The heart weight exceeded 400 g in 108 and 500 g in 42 patients.

In patients with heart muscle disease, between 40 and 60 per cent give a history indicating alcohol abuse.[21,22] AHMD is usually underdiagnosed in the hospital population and surveys have shown that 15–20 per cent of medical in-patients may give a history of alcohol abuse.

PATHOGENIC MECHANISMS

The direct toxic effect of alcohol on the heart has been established both in the experimental animal[23,24] and in man.[25–27] The effect of alcohol, however, will vary depending upon previous exposure and the presence of pre-existing cardiac disease. The effect of alcohol on the heart appears to relate to the blood alcohol, and the myocardial depression produced is reversible within a few hours.[26] In chronic alcoholics larger doses are required to produce an effect.[25,28] However, once an attack of heart failure or other cardiac complication has occurred further exposure to alcohol is likely to produce a similar response more readily.[26,29]

In order to understand the pathogenesis of alcoholic heart disease it is proposed to review the metabolic and pathological effects of alcohol on the heart and the myocardium in particular. These will then be related to the clinical pattern, investigations and management of the patient with alcoholic heart disease.

Myocardial Metabolic Effects

Acute

Acute alcohol exposure contributes to depression of the myocardial function which may be explained on a metabolic basis. In particular, there may be a response to an effect on calcium movement[30] or from changes in calcium flux at the microsomal level.[31] There are, furthermore, alterations in the active transport of potassium and sodium across the cell membrane, as suggested by Kalant and Israel.[32] This appears to be a basic mechanism of the effect of alcohol on any cell, not only the myocardial cell. In high doses alcohol may produce a transient loss of potassium and phosphate out of the muscle cell.

Alterations in lipid transport in the myocardium are now well recognized since Regan et al.[25] showed that alcohol reduced the uptake of free fatty acids (FFA) by the left ventricle. The increased triglyceride uptake that results promotes accumulation of the lipid in the myocardium. Using histopathological techniques Ferrans et al.[33] demonstrated substantial lipid deposits in the alcoholic heart. The reduced extraction of free fatty acids may relate to reduced arterial level of substrate as well as from competitive inhibition from increased extraction of acetate.

Further metabolic consequences of alcohol ingestion include increased production of lactate and acetate with increased utilization of these substrates by the heart.[34] It has also been found that the chronic intake of large amounts of alcohol results in a leakage of isocitrate and malic dehydrogenase into the coronary sinus regardless of the presence of clinical heart disease. Simultaneous decrease of FFA extraction occurs without alteration in the triglyceride extraction.[34]

It has been suggested that the toxic metabolites of alcohol, particularly acetaldehyde, are important in the pathogenesis of the myocardial damage[37] and that, in addition, a direct release of noradrenalin from the myocardium may further accentuate the myocardial changes.[38] Furthermore, acetaldehyde has been shown to affect the mitochondrial membranes and mitochondrial function[39] and also myocardial protein synthesis.[40,41]

Chronic

Although it is possible to demonstrate acute effects of alcohol on the myocardium the relationship of these to the pathogenesis of the clinical cardiac disease is less clear. It has indeed been suggested that at least 10 years of chronic alcohol exposure is required before the development of alcoholic heart muscle disease.[42] Therefore other workers have directed their attention to the effects of prolonged alcohol exposure on the myocardium.

Alcohol has been found to have an effect on the contractile proteins and their regulatory enzymes. It may also bring about an alteration in glycoprotein metabolism. An Alcian positive staining material may be detected in the muscle.[43]

Extracellular accumulation of sodium and water has been demonstrated using chromium 51 EDTA but there was no change in the potassium content.[44] It is possible that this effect results from an alteration in the membrane phospholipid concentration which thus limits the entrance of sodium and water into the cell. Increased sarcolemmal-myofibrillar distance has been observed in electron microscopic studies.[45] It has been suggested that these changes may limit the availability of calcium to the contractile proteins.

The experimental changes that have been observed closely resemble the myocardial damage which is seen in pre-clinical alcoholic heart disease in the human.[46-48]

PHYSIOLOGICAL EFFECTS OF ALCOHOL

Experimental

Exposure of rats to 25 per cent ethyl alcohol can be shown to produce depression of the peak isometric systolic tension.[49] Increased myocardial irritability and disturbances of cardiac rhythm were also noted in the same studies. More recently it has been shown in dogs that alcohol (36 per cent of total daily calorie intake) when given short term (18 months) and long term (52 months) would cause an increase in the left ventricular end diastolic pressure which was associated with an increase of the end diastolic and decrease in stroke volume.[44] However, when the velocity of the contractile element (used as an index of LV contractility) was measured the changes were only significant in the group which had had long-term exposure. The authors suggested that the altered contractility related to the availability of calcium to the contractile proteins.

Human

Acute administration of alcohol in normal man produces an increase in cardiac output and heart rate without altering the stroke volume.[50] The effect of alcohol on the submaximal exercise test is insignificant but myocardial oxygen consumption increases, possibly indicating a reduction of mechanical efficiency.[51] Similarly, in patients with fatty livers alcohol induces a depression of LV function with an increase in the left ventricular end diastolic pressure and a decrease in stroke work in response to increased aortic pressure.[52] Similarly, diminished ventricular performance in response to exercise has been observed in cirrhotic patients without evidence of cardiac disease.[47] Non-invasive systolic time interval studies in asymptomatic alcoholic subjects have shown some impairment of LV function.[46,48] A schematic representation of the various pathogenic mechanisms for the effects of alcohol and acetaldehyde on the myocardium is shown in *Figure 3*.

PATHOLOGY

At necropsy of patients with AHMD the heart is indistinguishable from dilated (congestive) cardiomyopathy with dilatation of both ventricular chambers.[53,54] The myocardium is pale and flabby with areas of diffuse fibrosis. Thrombus formation is often present when the chambers are dilated. The valves are normal except when there is functional dilatation of the mitral ring which may result in subvalvar mitral regurgitation.

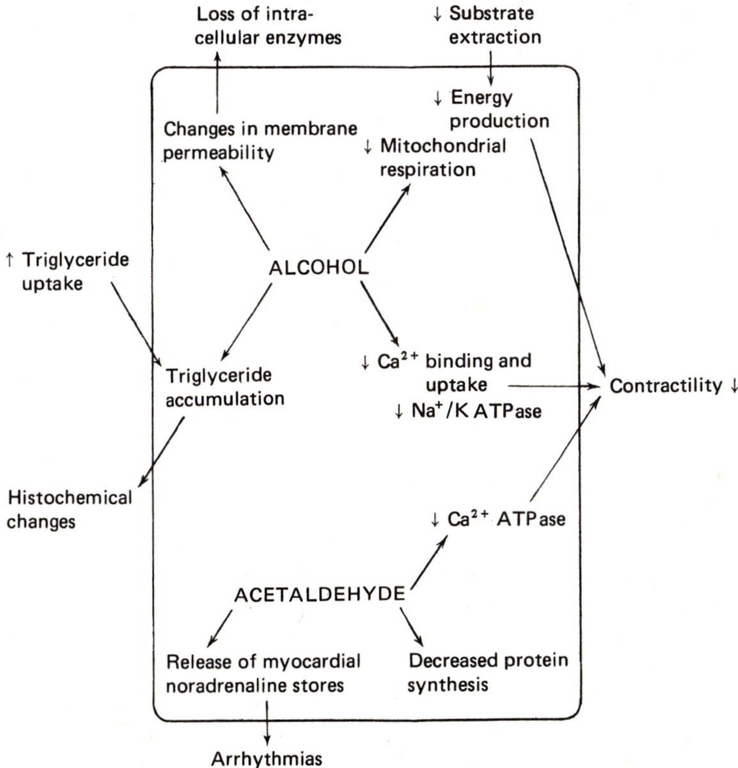

Figure 3. Suggested pathogenic mechanisms for action of alcohol on myocardium.

Histology

The histological findings are similar to those of a dilated cardiomyopathy.[55] The myocardial fibres are hypertrophied and may be attenuated when long-standing dilatation of the ventricles has been present. Some fraying of the myocardial fibres may also be present and occasional foci of inflammatory cells are seen. The latter findings do not necessarily imply the presence of a viral myocarditis. Indeed we have noted a Coxsackie virus neutralization titre suggestive of viral infection in only 1 out of 15 patients with AHMD. Interstitial fibrosis is a prominent feature, particularly at this late stage. Attenuation is not always seen even when the LV chamber is dilated. The coronary arteries are usually conspicuously normal. Factor[56] has, however, described intramyocardial small vessel disease in the alcoholic heart. The results of histopathological examination of the myocardial biopsies from 15 patients with AHMD are shown in Table 2. The

Table 2
Alcoholic heart disease—histological changes

Patient	*Endocardial/smooth muscle changes*	*Hypertrophy and regular arrangement*	*Attenuation*	*Fibrosis*	*Interstitial widening*	*Cellular infiltration*
WK	±	+	−	++	+	+
TO'D	−	+	−	±	+	+
HU	++	+	−	++	+	+
JB	±	+	−	++	−	±
AM	++	+	−	++	+	+
JU	±+	+	+	+±	−	+
JS	++	+	−	++	+	+
MH	++	+	−	++	−	+
CR	++	++	−	++	+	+
FS	±	+	−	±	−	+
LB	+	+	−	+	+	+
MR	±	+	−	++	−	−
GP	±	+	−	+	−	−
FC	++	+	+	−	+	±
SC	++	+	+	+	−	−

Reproduced by kind permission of Dr. E.G.J. Olsen.

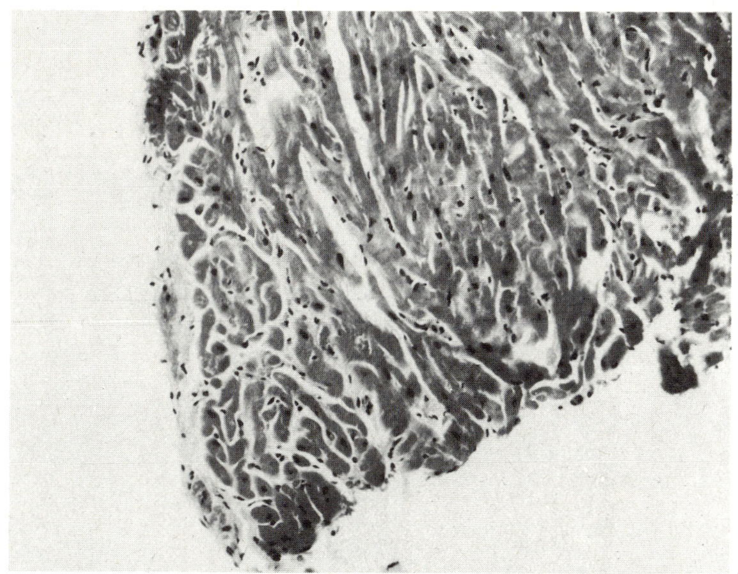

Figure 4. Light microscopic examination of a myocardial biopsy from patient with AHMD (HE stain magnification × 200), showing hypertrophied regularly arranged films without attenuation, some cellular infiltration and interstitial fibrosis. (Reproduced by kind permission of Dr. E.G.J. Olsen.)

histopathological details of a myocardial biopsy from a patient are shown in *Figure 4*.

Histochemistry

Large amounts of neutral lipid material may be deposited within the myocardial fibres as droplets 0·1–3·0 µm diameter.[33] The lipid deposits are mainly composed of triglycerides. The concentration of acid phosphatase positive lipofuscin granules is increased. Myocardial oxidative enzymes may be decreased, e.g. succinic dehydrogenase, lactate dehydrogenase and malic dehydrogenase.

Electron Microscopy

Whilst Alexander[45] described changes which he considered specific for alcoholic heart disease, these have now been found in dilated cardiomyopathy. The changes described include mitochondrial swelling, fragmentation of the cristae, swelling of the sarcoplasmic reticulum and varying degrees of myofibrillar disruption. Lysosomes and lipofuscin granules are scattered in large numbers throughout the myocardium.

These changes have been described in detail by Hibbs et al.[57] Furthermore, acute ultrastructural alterations have been shown in serial biopsies following intravenous infusion of alcohol.[58] An example of an electron micrograph from a patient with AHMD is shown in *Figure 5*, in which some of the features described above are detailed.

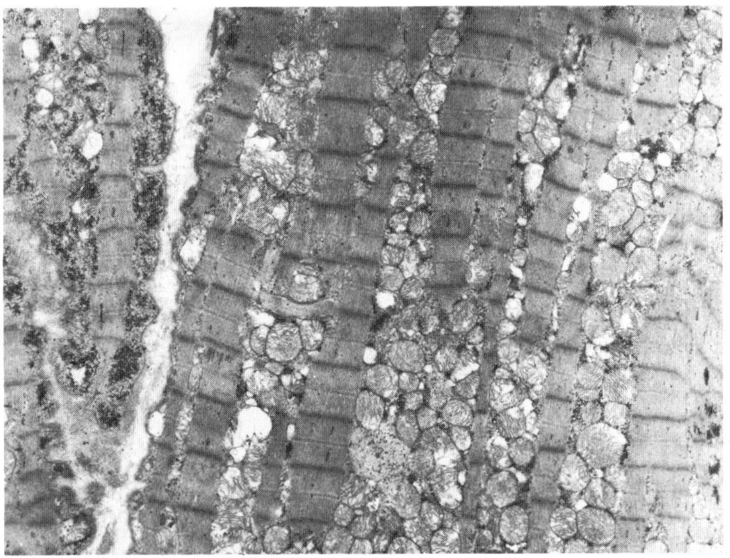

Figure 5. Electron micrograph of myocardial biopsy from a patient with AHMD. (Magnification × 9440.) (Reproduced by kind permission of Dr. E.G.J. Olsen.)

CLINICAL PRESENTATION

The usual presentation is with either heart failure or, perhaps less frequently, a symptomatic arrhythmia. The condition predominantly affects males in their fourth to sixth decades. With the recent change in drinking habits amongst women it is suspected that there may be an increase in alcohol-related cardiac problems.

The early diagnosis of alcoholic heart disease is particularly important since at this time the myocardial changes are likely to be reversible. In the early stage the usual presentation is with a history of palpitations. This is due to atrial arrhythmias or multiple ventricular premature beats. Atrial arrhythmias include paroxysmal or established atrial fibrillation or flutter. The episodic arrhythmias have been labelled the 'holiday heart syndrome' since they frequently result from bouts of heavy drinking.[59] Early alcoholic heart disease may present with features which mimic hyperthyroidism. The main signs relate to apparent sympathetic over-activity, namely tachycardia, sweating and tremor. Mild to moderate hypertension may be found on screening.

Whilst it is still possible that the patient may present at a later stage with an arrhythmia, it is more likely that the problem will relate to the consequences of myocardial damage. The main complaints therefore will be those of biventricular failure, namely exertional dyspnoea, orthopnoea, palpitation and even paroxysmal nocturnal dyspnoea. Oedema of the extremities and abdominal swelling may occur. Chest pain is a fairly frequent complaint and, contrary to previous experience, it is not infrequently of anginal type. Indeed in the latter context the patient may be admitted to the coronary care unit. In this situation it should be remembered that liver damage will cause a rise in the LDH and AST activity and that damage to skeletal muscle causes a rise in the CPK activity. The measurement of the CPK–MB activity will overcome this pitfall. Furthermore, studies have shown that between 1 and 10 per cent of patients admitted to hospital with a provisional diagnosis of infarction will have recently consumed alcohol to excess. A proportion of these patients, probably between 20 and 60 per cent, will have a raised CPK or AST, often to very high levels.[59a] The clinical findings may include an irregular pulse due to paroxysmal or established atrial fibrillation or multiple ventricular premature beats. The pulse pressure may narrow since the diastolic pressure is often raised. Whilst hypertension may be present initially the pressure may fall as myocardial failure develops. At this time the findings will include cardiomegaly and a palpable heart sound. Third and fourth heart sounds may be audible. A soft systolic murmur may reflect subvalvar mitral regurgitation. Signs of biventricular failure may be present. Stigmata of liver disease or alcohol disease are unusual, as is physical or psychological alcohol dependence.

INVESTIGATIONS

A reliable drinking history is difficult to obtain but it has been recently shown, using a structured interview, that exposure to alcohol can be ascertained with a high degree of reproducibility and reliability. This technique, based on the practice of obtaining a history of alcohol consumption related to key life events, offers the possibility of correctly estimating the quantity of alcohol consumed on a daily basis (submitted for publication) (see Table 1 for alcohol content of beverages). This may then be correlated with the degree and the nature of the target organ damage.

In order to clarify the safe limits of drinking with respect to myocardial disease, we are undertaking a study of drinking habits in patients who present with dilated cardiomyopathy. The history is taken without knowledge of the diagnosis which is established on clinical, angiographic and biopsy criteria (including myocardial enzyme activities).[60] The preliminary results of our study are shown in *Figure 6*.

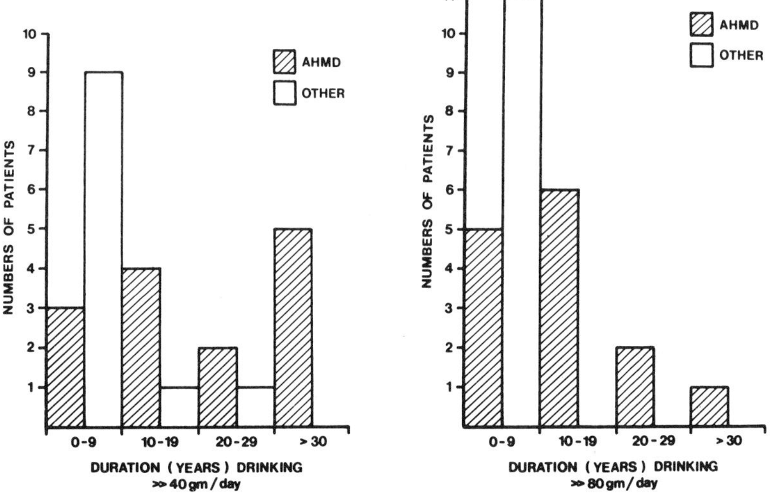

Figure 6. Analysis of drinking histories of patients presenting with dilated cardiomyopathy.

Analysis of the drinking histories shows that these fall into two clear groups. Among 14 patients with AHMD, 11 had consumed more than 40 g of alcohol a day for more than 10 years compared to only 2 out of 11 patients with cardiomyopathy of other causes. At the time of presentation alcohol consumption exceeded 40 g a day in 13 out of 14 patients with AHMD but reached this level in only 2 of 11 patients with cardiomyopathy. The lifetime alcohol intake also showed an impressive difference with 12 out of 14 AHMD patients exceeding 500 kg of alcohol, but only 1 out of 11 patients with cardiomyopathy exceeded this figure (see *Figure 7*).

These results suggest that, although there is some overlap, drinking habits of patients with AHMD differ markedly from patients with cardiomyopathy or other causes. Furthermore, increased risk of myocardial damage is evident at levels of 40–80 g of alcohol per day, which is not usually considered to be hazardous drinking.

Laboratory Tests

The combination of an elevated mean corpuscular volume of the erythrocyte (MCV) and a raised gamma glutamyl transpeptidase is a strong pointer to excessive alcohol consumption. Further indicators may include an elevated uric acid or triglyceride. Confirmation of suspected alcohol abuse may be substantiated by urinary or blood alcohol estimations.

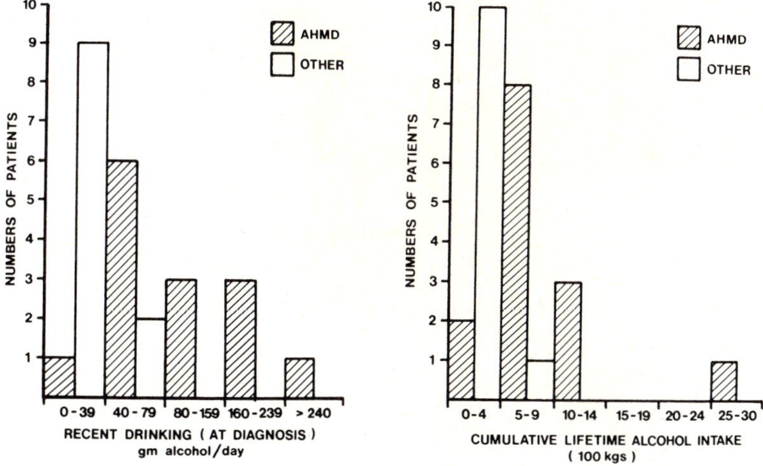

Figure 7. Lifetime cumulative alcohol intake in patients with cardiomyopathy and AHMD.

Cardiovascular Investigations

Electrocardiography

There are no pathognomonic changes in the electrocardiogram in alcoholic heart disease, although Evans[61] did suggest that the T wave might show a bifid or cloven pattern. In addition there may be atrio-ventricular conduction disturbances, bundle branch block and left ventricular hypertrophy.[62] The non-specific changes in the T waves and the ST segments may revert after the withdrawal of alcohol.

Chest Radiography

The most frequent finding on the chest X-ray is that of cardiomegaly. The cardiac enlargement may be found to regress following cessation of alcohol abuse. The other radiological findings relate to the presence of biventricular failure. An example of a patient admitted in failure and subsequently showing diminution of cardiomegaly is shown following 2 months' abstinence from alcohol (*Figure 8*).

Echocardiography

Whilst ECG and X-ray may reflect the late stage of the disease it appears that the echocardiogram may be able to detect the preclinical stage. In a detailed study by Matthews et al.[63] it was concluded that in symptomatic patients there was a decrease in the LV fractional fibre

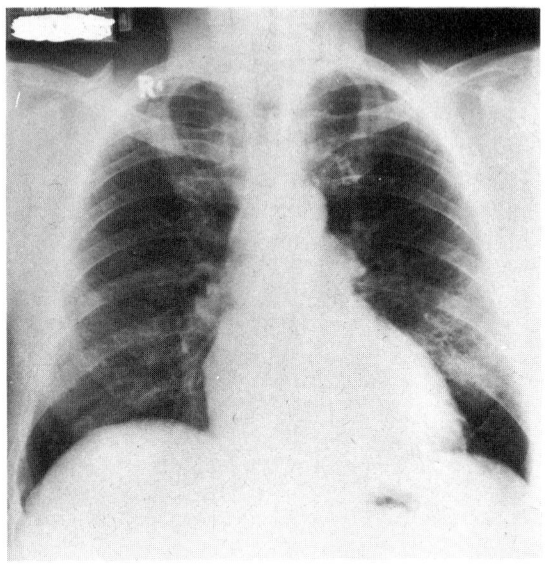

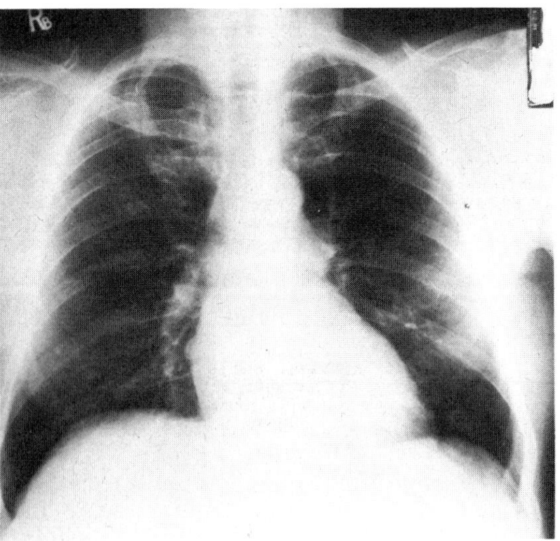

Figure 8. Chest radiographs showing 3 cm reduction of heart size and resolution of pulmonary congestion in a patient with AHMD following 2 months' abstinence.

shortening with significant increases in the LV systolic and diastolic dimensions. The LV mass and the left atrial dimensions were also increased. Similarly, there was an increase in at least one of these latter variables in 68 per cent of the asymptomatic group. They concluded that the echo was a useful means of detecting preclinical disease. Similar studies were also performed by Askanas et al.[64] who similarly found evidence of left ventricular hypertrophy and impaired contractility. These authors also confirmed the findings of Spodick et al.[46] with respect to the prolonged pre-ejection period, shortened ejection time and the increased PEP/LVET ratio.

A further non-invasive means of assessing the heart in alcoholic heart disease is by means of gated blood pool. This enables serial measurement of LV function not only after stress, such as isometric exercise or the cold pressor test, but also to determine the change after abstinence.[65]

INVASIVE ASSESSMENT OF ALCOHOLIC HEART DISEASE

The haemodynamic and the angiographic findings are, like the pathological changes, similar to those of congestive (dilated) cardiomyopathy. In the stage before the onset of myocardial failure the cardiac output may be normal or increased. The latter may result from the decreased peripheral resistance.[22]

Left ventricular angiography confirms the presence of some degree of left ventricular hypertrophy and this may be present before the development of ventricular dilatation and/or impairment of LV function. Mild to moderate mitral regurgitation may be demonstrated when the cavity dilatation is marked. In the majority of patients the coronary arteries are normal although minor degrees of atheroma may be found. *Figure 9* shows LV angiograms in systole and diastole of a patient with AHMD demonstrating poor contraction. The coronary arteries were normal.

The development of endomyocardial biopsy has facilitated the study of the myocardium from patients with suspected specific heart muscle disease. Small samples of right or left ventricular tissue of 3–5 mg wet weight may be excised at the time of cardiac catheterization. These samples may then be examined by histopathological, electron microscopical, virological and biochemical methods.

Examination of Myocardial Biopsy Samples

In addition to the haemodynamic and angiographic studies, routine endomyocardial biopsy may also be performed. Histopathological

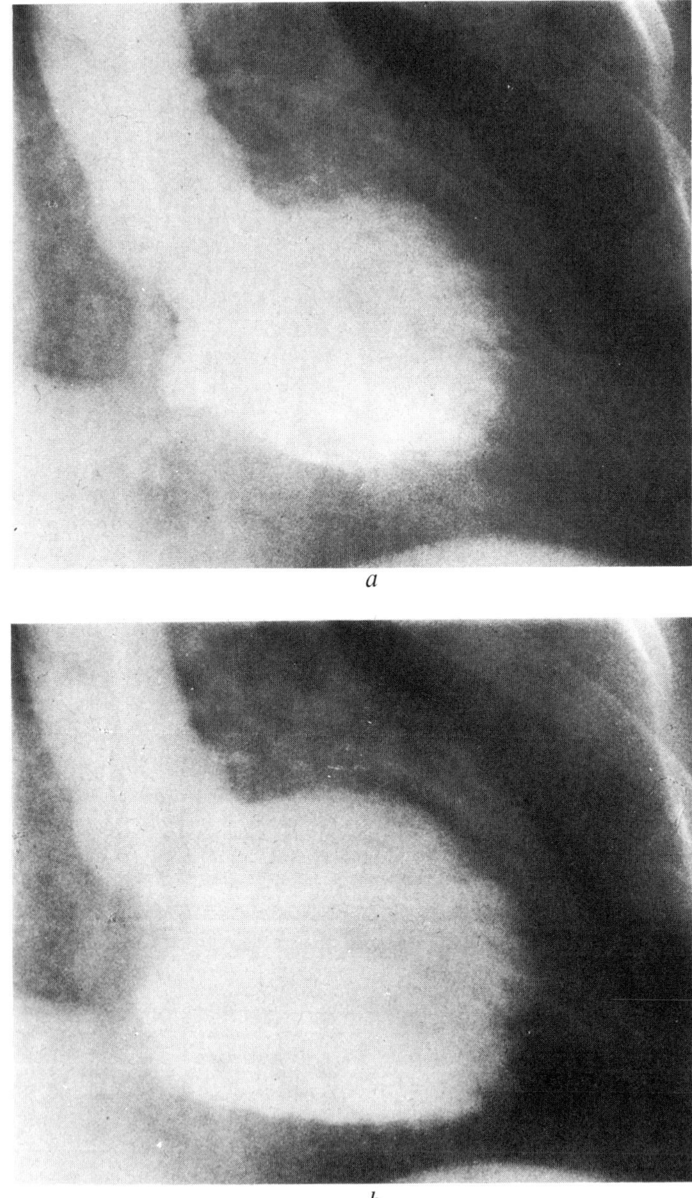

a

b

Figure 9. Left ventricular angiograms in systole (a) and diastole (b) (ejection fraction 38 per cent) from patient with AHMD whose chest radiographs are reproduced in Figure 8.

findings are similar to those in dilated cardiomyopathy. The results of the histopathological examination in 15 patients that were investigated for suspected AHMD are seen in Table 2.

In summary the findings were those of regularly arranged hypertrophied myocardial fibres without attenuation. Thickening of the endocardium and smooth muscle hypertrophy are usually present. Widening of the interstitium was not pronounced but interstitial fibrosis was a prominent feature. It is important to note that cellular infiltrates are a frequent finding but in these patients were not accompanied by positive virology. This may suggest that the appearances relate to the toxic effect of alcohol on the myocardium. At the present time we do not have data collected from patients biopsied serially after abstention. We have observed no evidence of disease in the small coronary vessels in AHMD.

Myocardial enzyme activities have been measured in different forms of cardiomyopathy in order to determine whether an alcohol characteristic diagnostic enzyme profile might be able to distinguish cryptogenic dilated cardiomyopathy from AHMD.[60,66] In order to clarify this point two groups of patients were taken: those drinking at the time of investigation (see Table 3a) and those who had stopped drinking 3 months prior to biopsy (see Table 3b). Whilst there was a clear

Table 3
(a) Enzyme activities in idiopathic COCM and COCM with alcohol excess

	Enzyme activities (mU/mg protein)					
	CPK	LDH	MDH	HBD	GOT	ICDH
Idiopathic COCM	1559	632	1586	471	500	45·8
n = 9	±188	±62	±193	±43·5	±65	±6·3
Alcohol excess	2189	922	2331	721	608	54·1
n = 9	±210	±75	±199	±67	±58	±9·1
p	0·05	0·01	0·05/0·2	0·02/0·01	ns	ns

Values are mean ± S.E.M.

Table 3
(b) Enzyme activities in COCM with alcohol excess and COCM with past alcohol

	Enzyme activities (mU/mg protein)					
	CPK	LDH	MDH	HBD	GOT	ICDH
Alcohol excess	2189	922	2331	721	608	54·1
n = 9	±210	±75	±199	±67	±58	±9·1
Past alcohol	1487	686	1728	517	275	48·9
n = 4	±185	±37	±58	±26	±56	±8·4
p	0·05	ns	ns	ns	0·05/0·02	ns

Values are mean ± S.E.M.

separation between idiopathic dilated cardiomyopathy and the AHMD group in those who had abstained, only the CPK and the GOT were significantly lower ($p < 0{\cdot}05$).

DIAGNOSIS

AHMD should be considered in the differential diagnosis of any patient presenting with dilated cardiomyopathy, but especially in Caucasian, middle-aged males. There are no diagnostic findings on examination and it is unusual for these patients to have signs of chronic liver disease or indeed other alcohol-related disease. Although an elevated gamma-glutamyl transpeptidase and mean corpuscular volume are supportive evidence of excessive consumption of alcohol, normal results are frequently seen in heavy drinkers. The importance of a detailed drinking history, taking particular note of the duration of drinking, consumption at presentation and lifetime consumption, is emphasized. Whilst the histological changes are similar to dilated cardiomyopathy the measurement of tissue enzyme activities in suspected AHMD may enable confirmation of the diagnosis.

TREATMENT

Since the effects of alcohol upon the myocardium are reversible in the early stage it is clearly important to be able to make an early diagnosis. It has already been emphasized that the detailed drinking history is important but other complementary investigations will include echocardiography if not the routine use of myocardial biopsy. If the disease can be diagnosed before the onset of frank cardiac failure the single most important measure is to obtain complete abstinence. If the disease is suspected at a later stage when atrial fibrillation or radiological evidence of cardiomegaly has supervened, the outcome is less predictable. Certainly, however, following complete withdrawal from alcohol even at this point, as we have seen, there may be a dramatic improvement. When this measure is ineffective the standard measures to treat the heart failure should be used. These will include digitalis and diuretics with careful monitoring of the electrolytes.

In those patients in whom there is a poor response to diuretic therapy the use of vasodilator therapy may be beneficial, as indeed it is in other patients with cardiomyopathy. The choice of drugs includes prazosin, hydrallazine or the nitrates. The effects of these drugs, however, have not been specifically investigated in patients with AHMD nor indeed has the effect of beta-blockade which has been shown to be beneficial in some patients with dilated cardiomyopathy.

It has been suggested by Burch et al.[23] that a period of prolonged bed rest may be therapeutic. Indeed, they reported that in a series of 48 patients with alcoholic cardiomyopathy following bed rest 21 (44 per cent) had a normal heart size and an absence of symptoms, 11 (23 per cent) lost their symptoms without a complete reduction in the heart size, 5 (10 per cent) had no reduction in the heart size but improved clinically, 4 (8 per cent) died during the initial period of bed rest and 7 patients discharged themselves against advice.[21] In the long term (6·25 years) 13 (62 per cent) whose hearts had returned to normal size were still alive and, of these, 9 (43 per cent) still had a normal heart size. Four (36 per cent), who had had a partial reduction in the size of the heart, and 3 (60 per cent), who had shown no change in the cardiomegaly, were still alive with enlarged hearts.

The clinical impression that in alcoholic heart muscle disease (AHMD) improvement in the cardiac function will follow abstention from alcohol is further supported by the observations of Schwarz et al.[67] They found that improvement in the indices of ventricular function occurred and were maintained during an 18-month follow-up. Similarly, Hung et al.[65] observed a similar improvement following abstinence which was monitored by gated blood pool scanning. The clinical implications of these studies are obvious but are perhaps of great interest since the improvement followed abstention and did not require prolonged bed rest to achieve an effect.

CONCLUSION

Alcohol abuse is an important cause of heart muscle disease and the recent worldwide increase in alcohol consumption can be expected to result in an increasing incidence of this problem.

The patient is usually a middle-aged male presenting with cardiac failure or an arrhythmia, and there are usually no diagnostic findings on examination. Laboratory screening tests may provide evidence which suggest alcohol abuse and a detailed drinking history should be taken to confirm the clinical impression. This will usually reveal a pattern of consumption exceeding 40 g/day for more than 10 years. The diagnosis of AHMD can now be confirmed by myocardial enzyme analysis, with histological, histochemical and ultrastructural changes indistinguishable from dilated cardiomyopathy.

Experimental work on animals and human data are providing insight into the complex mechanisms of impaired myocardial function and subsequent damage.

The prognosis following abstention from alcohol is very encouraging and justifies careful supervision of such patients to promote the achievement of total abstinence. Patients with AHMD are usually heavy social drinkers, not physically or psychologically dependent on alcohol, and can often be persuaded to abstain without difficulty.

ACKNOWLEDGEMENTS

One of the authors (PJR) wishes to acknowledge the support of Merck Sharp and Dohme International Research, Joint Research Trust, King's College Hospital and the British Heart Foundation for his metabolic and virological studies in cardiomyopathy.

REFERENCES

1. Schmidt W. In: Edwards G, Grant M, eds. *Cirrhosis and alcohol consumption: an epidemiological perspective in alcoholism: new knowledge and responses*. London: Croom Helm, 1977: 15.
2. Royal College of Psychiatry. *Report of a special committee on alcohol and alcoholism*. London: Tavistock, 1979.
3. Pequignot L, Chabret G, Ieydoux N, Courcout MA. Increased risk of cirrhosis in relation to consumption of alcohol. *Rev Alcool* 1974; **20**: 191.
4. Wilson P. *Drinking in England and Wales*. Office of Population, Census, and Surveys. London: HMSO, 1980.
5. Goodwin JF, Oakley CM. The cardiomyopathies. *Br. Heart J* 1972; **34**: 545.
6. Report of the WHO/ISFC task force on the definition and classification of the cardiomyopathies. *Br Heart J* 1980; **44**: 672.
7. Brigden W, Robinson J. Alcoholic heart disease. *Br Med J* 1964; **2**: 1283.
8. McIntyre N, Stanley NN. Cardiac beri-beri: two modes of presentation. *Br Med J* 1971; **3**: 567–9.
9. Sambrook PN, Dalton WR. Shoshin beri-beri. *Aust NZ J Med* 1981; **11**: 190–2.
10. Alexander CS. Cobalt-beer cardiomyopathy. A clinical and pathological study of 28 cases. *Am J Med* 1972; **53**: 395.
11. Lian C. L'alcoolisme cause d'hypertension arterielle. *Bull Acad Med (Paris)* 1915; **74**: 525.
12. Klatsky AL, Friedman GD, Sieglaub AB, Gerard MJ. Alcohol consumption and blood pressure. *N Engl J Med* 1977; **296**: 1194.
13. Ramsay LE. Liver dysfunction in hypertension. *Lancet* 1977; **2**: 111.

13a. Beevers DG. Alcohol and hypertension *Lancet* 1977; **2**: 114.

14. Ashley MJ, Rankin DG. Alcohol consumption—evidence from hazardous drinking and alcoholic populations. *Aust NZ J Med* 1979; **9**: 201.
15. Klatsky AL, Friedman GD, Sieglaub AB. Alcohol consumption before myocardial infarction. *Ann Intern Med* 1974; **81**: 294.
16. Marmot MG, Rose G, Shipley MJ, Rhomas B. Alcohol and mortality: a U-shaped curve. *Lancet* 1981; **1**: 580.
17. Turner T, Bennett VL, Hernandez H. The beneficial side of moderate alcohol use. *Johns Hopkins Med J* 1981; **148**: 53.
18. Schmidt W, Popham RE. The role of drinking and smoking in mortality from cancer. *Cancer* 1981; **47**: 1031–41.
19. Schenk EA, Cohen J. The heart in chronic alcoholism: clinical and pathological findings. *Pathol Microbiol* 1970; **35**: 96.
20. Morgan RR. Heart disease and alcoholism. *Circulation* 1961; **24**: 1001.
21. McDonald CD, Burch GE, Walsh JJ. Alcoholic cardiomyopathy and prolonged bed rest. *Ann Intern Med* 1971; **74**: 681.
22. Masummi RA, Rias JC, Gooch AS, Nutter D, De Vita VT, Datlow DW. Primary myocardial disease: report of 50 cases and review of the subject. *Circulation* 1965; **31**: 19.
23. Burch GE, Colcolough HL, Harb HM, Tsui CY. The effect of the ingestion of ethyl alcohol, wine and beer on the myocardium in mice. *Am J Cardiol* 1971; **27**: 522.

24. Vasdec SC, Chakavarti RN, Subrahmanyam D, Jain AC, Wahi PL. Myocardial lesions induced by prolonged alcohol feeding in rhesus monkeys. *Cardiovasc Res* 1975; **9**: 134.
25. Regan TJ, Kuroxenidis GT, Moschos CB, Oldewurtel HA, Lehan PH, Hellems HK. The acute metabolic and haemodynamic response of the left ventricle to ethanol. *J Clin Invest* 1966; **45**: 270.
26. Regan TJ. Ethyl alcohol and the heart. *Circulation* 1971; **44**: 957.
27. Friedman HS, Lieber CS. Cardiotoxicity of alcohol. *Cardiovasc Med* 1977; **2**: 111.
28. Wong M. Depression of cardiac performance by ethanol unmasked during autonomic blockade. *Am Heart J* 1973; **86**: 508.
29. Timmis GC, Ramos RG, Gorden S, Gangadharan V. The basis for the differences in ethanol-induced myocardial depression in normal subjects. *Circulation* 1975; **51**: 1144.
30. Seeman P, Chan M, Goldberg M, Sanks T, Sax L, The binding of Ca^{2+} to cell membrane increased by volatile anaesthetics (alcohol, acetone, ether) which induce sensitisation of nerve or muscle. *Biochim Biophys Acta* 1971; **225**: 185.
31. Retig JN, Kirchberger MA, Rubin E, Katz AM. Effects of alcohol on calcium transport by microsomes phosphorylated by cyclic AMP dependent protein kinase. *Biochem Pharmacol* 1977; **26**: 393.
32. Kalant H, Israel Y. Effects of ethanol on active transport of cations. In: Maiskel RP, ed. *Biochemical factors in alcohol.* Oxford: Pergamon Press, 1967: 25.
33. Ferrans VJ, Hibbs RG, Weilbacher DG, Black WC, Walsh JJ, Burch GE. Alcoholic cardiomyopathy: a histochemical study. *Am Heart J* 1965; **69**: 748.
34. Lindeneg O, Mellangaard K, Fabricius J, Lindquist F. Myocardial utilisation of acetate, lactate, FFA after ingestion of ethanol. *Clin Sci* 1964; **27**: 427.
35. Wendt VF, Wu C, Balcon R, Doty C, Bing RJ. Haemodynamic and metabolic effects of chronic alcoholism in man. *Am J Cardiol* 1965; **15**: 175.
36. Wendt VE, Ajluni R, Bruce TA, Prasad AS, Bing RJ. Acute effects of alcohol on the human myocardium. *Am J Cardiol* 1966; **17**: 804.
37. Kikuchi T, Kako KJ. Metabolic effects of ethanol on the rabbit heart. *Circulation Res* 1970; **26**: 625.
38. James TN, Bear ES. Effects of ethanol and acetaldehyde on the heart. *Am Heart J* 1977; **74**: 243.
39. Rubin E, Beattie DS, Lieber CS. Effects of ethanol on the biogenesis of mitochondrial membranes and associated mitochondrial functions. *Lab Invest* 1970; **23**: 620.
40. Schreiber SS, Brigden K, Oratz M, Rothschild MA. Ethanol, acetaldehyde and myocardial protein synthesis. *J Clin Invest* 1972; **51**: 2820.
41. Schreiber SS, Oratz M, Rothschild MA. Alcoholic cardiomyopathy II. The inhibition of cardiac microsomal protein synthesis by acetaldehyde. *J Mol Cell Cardiol* 1974; **6**: 207.
42. Levi GF, Quadri A, Ratti S, Basagni M. Preclinical abnormality of left ventricular function in chronic alcoholics. *Br Heart J* 1977; **39**: 35.
43. Regan TJ, Khan MI, Ettinger PO, Haider B, Lyons MM, Oldewurtel HA. Myocardial function and lipid metabolism in the chronic alcoholic animal. *J Clin Invest* 1974; **54**: 740.
44. Thomas G, Haider B, Oldewurtel HA, Lyons MM, Yeh CK, Regan TJ. Progression of myocardial abnormalities in experimental alcoholism. *Am J Cardiol* 1980; **46**: 233.
45. Alexander CS. Electron microscopic observations in alcoholic heart disease. *Br Heart J* 1967; **29**: 200.
46. Spodick DH, Pigott VM, Chirife R. Preclinical cardiac malfunction in chronic alcoholism. Comparisons with matched normal controls and with alcoholic cardiomyopathy. *N Engl J Med* 1972; **287**: 677.
47. Gould L, Shariff M, Dilieto M. Cardiac haemodynamics in alcoholic patients with chronic liver disease and presystolic gallop. *J Clin Invest* 1969; **48**: 860.

48. Wu CF, Sudhakar M, Jafari G, Ahmed SS, Regan TJ. Preclinical cardiomyopathy in chronic alcoholics: a sex difference. *Am Heart J* 1976; **91**: 281.
49. Maines JE, Aldinger EE. Myocardial depression accompanying chronic consumption of alcohol. *Am Heart J* 1967; **73**: 55.
50. Riff DP, Jain AC, Doyle JT. Acute haemodynamic effects of ethanol on normal human volunteers. *Am Heart J* 1969; **78**: 592.
51. Mitchell JH, Cohen LS. Alcohol and the heart. *Mod Concepts Cardiovasc Dis* 1970; **39**: 109.
52. Regan TJ, Levinson GE, Oldewurtel HA, Frank MJ, Weisse AB, Moschos GB. Ventricular function in non-cardiacs with alcoholic fatty liver: role of ethanol in the production of cardiomyopathy. *J Clin Invest* 1969; **48**: 397.
53. Goodwin JF. Congestive and hypertrophic cardiomyopathies—a decade of study. *Lancet* 1970; **1**: 731.
54. Olsen EGJ. *The pathology of the heart*, 2nd ed. London: Macmillan, 1980.
55. Olsen EGJ. Pathological recognition of cardiomyopathy. *Postgrad Med J* 1975; **51**: 277.
56. Factor SM. Intramyocardial small vessel disease in chronic alcoholism. *Am Heart J* 1976, **92**: 561.
57. Hibbs RG, Ferrans VJ, Black WC, Weilbacher DC, Walsh JJ, Burch GE. Alcoholic cardiomyopathy—an electron microscopic study. *Am Heart J* 1965; **69**: 766.
58. Klein H, Harmjanz D. Effect of ethanol infusion on the ultrastructure of the human myocardium. *Postgrad Med J* 1975; **51**: 325.
59. Ettinger PO, Wu CF, De La Cruz C Jr, Woesse AB, Ahmed S, Regan TJ. Arrhythmias and the holiday heart. Alcohol associated cardiac rhythm disorders. *Am Heart J* 1978; **95**: 555.
59a Nevins MA, Saran M, Bright M, Lyon LJ. Pitfalls in interpreting serum creatinine phosphokinase activity. *JAMA* 1973; **224**: 1382.
60. Richardson PJ, Atkinson L. The measurement of enzyme activities in endomyocardial biopsy samples from patients with cardiomyopathy. In: Sekiguchi M, Olsen EGJ, eds. *Cardiomyopathy: clinical, pathological and theoretical aspects.* Tokyo: University of Tokyo Press, 1980: 149.
61. Evans W. The electrocardiogram of alcoholic cardiomyopathy. *Br Heart J* 1959; **21**: 445.
62. Bashour TT, Fahdul H, Cheng TO. Electrocardiographic abnormalities in alcoholic cardiomyopathy. A study in 65 patients. *Chest* 1973; **68**: 240.
63. Matthews EC, Gardin JM, Henry WL et al. Echocardiographic abnormalities in chronic alcoholics with and without overt congestive cardiac failure. *Am J Cardiol* 1981; **47**: 570.
64. Askanas A, Udoshi M, Sadjadi SA. The heart in chronic alcoholism; a non-invasive study. *Am Heart J* 1980; **99**: 9.
65. Hung J, Harris PJ, Kelly DT, Richmond DR, Hutton BF, Bartovich G. Improvement of left ventricular function in alcoholic cardiomyopathy documented by serial gated cardiac pool scanning. *Aust NZ J Med* 1979; **9**: 420.
66. Richardson PJ, Atkinson L, Oram S. Enzyme activities in endomyocardial biopsy samples from patients with cardiomyopathy (abstract). *Br Heart J* 1978; **40**: 456.
67. Schwartz L, Sample KA, Wigle ED. Severe alcoholic cardiomyopathy reversed with abstention from alcohol. *Am J Cardiol* 1975; **36**: 963.

Chapter 10

Drug toxicity and the heart: potential molecular mechanisms

Michael R. Bristow

This chapter is devoted to a brief discussion of drug-induced myocardial cytotoxicity. Several potentially important molecular mechanisms will be examined, in the context of which some clinical syndromes of drug-related cardiotoxicity will be discussed.

'CALCIUM OVERLOAD'

The function of the myocardium is continually and rhythmically to contract and relax, or to function as a pump. The mechanics of this are accomplished by rapid movements of cellular ionized calcium. Contraction is achieved when cytoplasmic Ca^{2+} reaches a critical concentration—that is, probably around 10 μM; relaxation occurs when the Ca^{2+} concentration near the myofilaments is reduced, probably to around 0·1 μM.[1] In myocardium the pool of Ca^{2+} available for coupling contraction is in rapid equilibrium with the extracellular space,[2,3] which has a Ca^{2+} in the mM range. Thus the myocardial cell must have mechanisms which can cope with Ca^{2+} gradients approaching four orders of magnitude, and must be capable of rapidly adjusting the cytoplasmic concentration over two orders of magnitude.

Myocardial Ca^{2+} homeostasis is maintained by specialized adaptations in the sarcolemma, sarcoplasmic reticulum, contractile proteins, and possibly in the mitochondria. These adaptations not only allow for the rapid Ca^{2+} movements that mediate contraction and relaxation, but also ensure that the intracellular Ca^{2+} level does not reach toxic levels.

There is ample evidence that Ca^{2+} and other extracellular cation translocations are extremely cytotoxic, and that they may be a 'final common pathway' for cell death.[4] As the heart is exquisitely dependent on Ca^{2+} homeostasis, it is not surprising that it would be highly susceptible to Ca^{2+}-mediated cytotoxicity. As elucidated by Fleckenstein,[5,6] cellular calcium 'overload' involves: (1) an increase in cytoplasmic Ca^{2+}, either by damage to cellular structures responsible for maintaining normal Ca^{2+} homeostasis or by 'pharmacological' increases, such as by catecholamines; and (2) exhaustion of high energy phosphates and a 'metabolic' form of cell injury and death brought about by the increase in intracellular Ca^{2+}.

There is good evidence for both tenets of the 'calcium overload' theory, and there is not much doubt of its importance as a final step in myocardial cytotoxicity. However, with the exception of catecholamine necrosis there is no good evidence implicating this mechanism as a primary lesion in drug-induced cytotoxicity, and even catecholamine necrosis has other pathogenetic explanations (see below).

FREE RADICAL FORMATION

The formation of highly reactive oxygen radicals, such as hydroxyl and superoxide ions and H_2O_2, is a known mechanism of cell injury.[7] Here the primary lesion may be lipid peroxidation-related membrane injury.[8] It may be that the mammalian heart is deficient in enzymatic mechanisms of radical 'scavenging', such as catalase and superoxide dismutase, and as such is predisposed to this kind of damage.[9] After membrane injury occurs further cell injury would then proceed via the 'calcium overload' pathway.

Of known cardiac toxins, there is evidence that anthracycline antibiotics, such as adriamycin, may produce myocardial injury by stimulating the formation of free radicals.[8] One strength of this putative mechanism of anthracycline cardiotoxicity is that it provides an explanation for the location of the primary lesion in the sarcoplasmic reticulum, where adriamycin has been shown to stimulate free radical formation.[10] A weakness of this hypothesis is that free radical scavengers have not proved to be protective against development of anthracycline cardiomyopathy in humans or animal models.[11,12]

VASCULAR (ISCHAEMIA)-MEDIATED MYOCARDIAL INJURY

One relatively new pathogenetic explanation for myocardial injury is through vasoconstriction and 'microvascular spasm'.[13] The heart is heavily dependent on aerobic metabolism, and the cytotoxic consequences of ischaemia are well-documented. Vasoconstriction may play a role in the pathogenesis of catecholamine necrosis, where the lesion is compatible with a micro-infarct. Other vasoactive agents that are known to produce myocardial damage via a vasoconstrictor mechanism are angiotensin[14] and histamine.[15] The latter is a potent vasoconstrictor in the coronary artery of rabbits[16] and humans[17] and can produce catecholamine-like myocardial damage when infused in high doses.[15] This damage is totally prevented by pretreatment with H_1 blocking agents, which prevent the coronary vasoconstriction (Kantrowitz and Bristow, unpublished data).

A recent study by Factor et al.[13] emphasizes the potential importance of microvascular spasm in producing myocardial injury. Utilizing a latex perfusion technique, these investigators documented foci of microvascular spasm in the Syrian golden hamster at a time just before myopathy spontaneously appears. It has been known for several years that calcium antagonists can delay the development of myopathy in this model, and it was assumed that this was secondary to prevention of calcium overload. Since calcium antagonists are potent inhibitors of coronary vasospasm, it is possible that the primary lesion in this 'classical' animal model of heart muscle disease is vascular rather than myocardial.

Additionally, there is evidence that other types of myocardial injury may be related to vasoconstriction and/or microvascular effects. The cardiomyopathy produced by the anti-cancer drug adriamycin can be prevented in animals by pharmacological antagonism of the effects of vasoactive substances (histamine, catecholamines and prostaglandins) that are released by the drug.[18,19] Whether these released agents exert their effects on the myocardium or the vasculature is not entirely known, but knowledge of their pharmacological activity would favour a vascular mechanism. The myopathic effects of vasoconstriction–small vessel spasm will undoubtedly receive more attention in the future.

NUTRITIONAL–METABOLIC CAUSES

There is good evidence that nutritional–metabolic causes may lead to myocardial disease. The demonstration that protein-calorie malnutrition may lead to cardiomyopathy in animals and humans[20] suggests that cellular mechanisms involving defective protein synthesis might be involved in the pathogenesis of myocardial disease. For example, myocardial proteins are in a dynamic state and turn over with half lives anywhere from a few hours to a few days. These proteins are used not only for contraction but to maintain the heart's sophisticated array of enzymatic and structural compounds. It is well known that drugs may influence the rate of degradation and synthesis of myocardial protein[21] and are thus in a position to affect heart muscle disease by this mechanism.

Recent work by Van Vleet, Ferrans and Ruth[22,23] illustrates that a defect in a trace mineral may lead to myocardial and vascular damage. The mechanism of this form of cytotoxicity apparently is through a deficiency of the selenoenzyme glutathione peroxidase, a free radical 'scavenger'. Thus free radical membrane damage and calcium overload enter into the distal components of this injury pathway.

VASOACTIVE SUBSTANCES AND ABNORMALITIES IN CELLULAR HORMONE RECEPTORS

Several endogenous vaso-cardioactive hormones are associated with the development of heart muscle disease. These include catecholamines,[24] thyroxine,[25] angiotensin,[14] histamine[15] and probably serotonin. Because of the 'physiological' presence of these potent hormones, homeostatic mechanisms have evolved that ordinarily ensure that toxic levels of each are not reached. For catecholamines these include neuronal and extra-neuronal uptake systems, and mechanisms for rapid metabolism. In the case of histamine there are uptake systems, metabolic pathways and release of 'physiological antagonists'.[26] Thyroxine levels are tightly regulated by feedback mechanisms involving the anterior pituitary.

There are, of course, examples of what may happen when these regulatory mechanisms fail, or when synthesis or release overwhelms hormone elimination. These include myocardial damage in patients with phaeochromocytoma, thyroid heart disease, the endocardial injury of carcinoid syndrome, and perhaps anthracycline cardiotoxicity.[18,19]

There are additional ways in which heart muscle damage might result from the effects of vaso-cardioactive substances, even when blood or tissue levels of these substances are in the 'physiological' range. Each hormone exerts its cellular effect by the following general pharmacological mechanism.

$$A+R \rightleftharpoons AR \longrightarrow 1 \longrightarrow 2 \longrightarrow n \longrightarrow \text{Effect}$$

'A' is a hormone 'agonist' that combines with a specific membrane receptor to produce a drug-receptor complex. The formation of this complex then either catalyses a subsequent enzymatic reaction (such as for catecholamines, thyroid hormone and histamine catalysing the activation of adenylate cyclase) or activates a calcium flux mechanism, such as with catecholamine, histamine or serotonin-induced coronary vascular contraction. In the heart '1' is therefore catalytic activation of adenylate cyclase, '2' is cyclic AMP, and the last step is calcium flux to the myofilaments. For human coronary artery vasoconstriction '1' is the activation of calcium pools,[27] and subsequent steps may involve phosphorylation and the calcium-binding protein calmodulin.[28] For both the coronary artery and myocardium 'effect' is muscle contraction.

The combination of agonist with receptor obeys mass action laws as applied to small molecules interacting with binding sites on larger molecules. It can be shown[29] that

$$E_A/E_M = f(S) = f(e \cdot y) = f\left(\frac{\{R\}_T K_A \{A\}}{\{RA\} + \{RA\} K_A}\right)$$

where E_A/E_M is response on a percentage of maximum basis, and S is the stimulus to the system imparted by the combination of drug with receptor. S can be subdivided into e, the efficacy of the drug, a linear component, and y, the proportion of receptor site occupied, a non-linear component. Through rearranging mass action equations $e \cdot y$ can be expressed in terms of the total number of receptors $\{R\}_T$, the affinity constant of the agonist, K_A, the agonist concentration $\{A\}$ and the number of agonist–receptor complexes $\{RA\}$. As can be seen from the above equation the response is thus proportional not only to the amount of agonist present, but also to the total number of receptors and the structural nature of the receptor, reflected by K_A. In other words, an increase in receptor density (up-regulation) or increase in receptor affinity (K_A) will accomplish the same purpose as increasing the concentration of agonist.

For the past several years our laboratory has been exploring the role of receptor regulation in heart muscle disease. Based on our own work, and the work of others, two conclusions have been reached: (1) conditions which cause up-regulation of receptors can be associated with subsequent vascular or myocardial tissue damage;[30-33] and (2) once heart muscle disease occurs, down-regulation of β-adrenergic receptors occurs, which imparts subsensitivity to the adrenergic pathway.[34]

In this chapter I have not attempted an extensive review of drug-induced heart disease, which is available elsewhere.[35] Rather, I have chosen to focus on several possible fundamental biological mechanisms of cardiac damage, all of which deserve additional investigation in the pathogenesis of heart muscle disease.

REFERENCES

1. Katz AM. *Physiology of the heart*. New York: Raven Press, 1977.
2. Bailey LE, Dresel PE. Correlation of contractile force with a calcium pool in the isolated cat heart. *J Gen Physiol* 1968; **52**: 969–83.

3. Shine KI, Serena SD, Langer GA. Kinetic localization of contractile calcium in rabbit myocardium. *Am J Physiol* 1971; **221**: 1408–17.
4. Schanne FAX, Kane AB, Young EE, Farber JL. Calcium dependence of toxic cell death: a final common pathway. *Science* 1979; **206**: 700–2.
5. Fleckenstein A, Janke J, Doering HJ, Pachinger O. Ca overload as the determinant factor in the production of catecholamine-induced myocardial lesions. *In*: Bajusz E, Rona E, eds. *Recent advances in studies on cardiac structure and metabolism*, vol. 2. Freiburg: Physiological Institute, University of Freiburg, 1973: 455–66.
6. Fleckenstein A, Janke J, Doering HJ, Leder O. Myocardial fiber necrosis due to intracellular Ca overload—a new principle in cardiac pathophysiology. In: Challas NS, ed. *Recent advances in studies on cardiac structure and metabolism*, vol. 4. Baltimore: University Park Press, 1974: 563–80.
7. Fridovich I. The biology of oxygen radicals. The superoxide radical is an agent of oxygen toxicity; superoxide dismutases provide an important defense. *Science* 1978; **201**: 875–80.
8. Myers CE, McGuire WP, Liss RH, Ifrim I, Grotzinger K, Young RC. Adriamycin: the role of lipid peroxidation in cardiac toxicity and tumour response. *Science* 1977; **197**: 165–7.
9. Doroshow JH, Locker GY, Myers CE. Enzymatic defenses of the mouse heart against reactive oxygen metabolites. *J Clin Invest* 1980; **65**: 128–35.
10. Doroshow JH, Reeves J. Daunorubicin-stimulated reactive oxygen metabolism in cardiac sarcosomes. *Biochem Pharmacol* 1981; **30**: 259–62.
11. Bristow MR. Anthracycline cardiotoxicity. In: Bristow MR, ed. *Drug-induced heart disease*. Amsterdam: Biomedical Press, 1980: 191–215.
12. Legha S, Benjamin R, Wang YM et al. Evaluation of α-tocopherol against adriamycin cardiotoxicity. (Abstract.) ASCO Proceedings, 1981. *ASCO Abstracts* 1981; **22**: 176.
13. Factor SM, Minase T, Okun EM, Herskowitz A, Sonnenblick EH. Coronary microvascular spasm in the cardiomyopathic Syrian hamster: a primary cause of focal cell necrosis? (Abstract.) *Circulation* 1980; **62**: suppl. III, III–254.
14. Ginsburg R, Bristow M, Kantrowitz NE. Histamine provocation of clinical coronary artery spasm: implications concerning pathogenesis of variant angina pectoris. *Am Heart J* 1981; **102**: 819–22.
15. Kantrowitz NE, Minobe WA, Bristow MR, Billingham ME. Histamine-mediated myocardial necrosis. (Abstract.) *Circulation* 1981; **64** (Suppl. 4): iv–282.
16. Coruzzi G, Bongrami S, Bertaccini G. Histamine receptors in the heart and coronary vessels of rabbits. *Pharmacol Res Commun* 1979; **11**: 517.
17. Ginsburg R, Bristow MR, Stinson EB, Harrison DC. Histamine receptors in the human heart. *Life Sci* 1980; **26**: 2245–9.
18. Bristow MR, Sageman WS, Scott RH et al. Acute and chronic cardiovascular effects of doxorubicin in the dog: the cardiovascular pharmacology of drug-induced histamine release. *J Cardiovasc Pharm* 1980; **2**: 487–515.
19. Bristow MR, Minobe WA, Billingham ME et al. Anthracycline-associated cardiac and renal damage in rabbits: evidence for mediation by vasoactive substances. *Lab Invest* 1981; **45**: 157–68.
20. Abel RM. Nutritional aspects of myocardial disease. In: Bristow MR, ed. *Drug-induced heart disease*. Amsterdam: Biomedical Press, 1980: 341–57.
21. Everett AW, Zak R. Protein synthesis and degradation in the normal and diseased myocardium. In: Bristow MR, ed. *Drug-induced heart disease*. Amsterdam: Biomedical Press, 1980: 63–80.
22. Van Vleet JF, Ferrans VJ, Ruth GR. Ultrastructural alterations in nutritional cardiomyopathy of selenium-vitamin E deficient swine. I. Fiber lesions. *Lab Invest* 1977; **37**: 188–200.

23. Van Vleet JF, Ferrans VJ, Ruth GR. Ultrastructural alterations in nutritional cardiomyopathy of selenium-vitamin E deficient swine. II. Vascular lesions. *Lab Invest* 1977; **37**: 201–11.
24. Rona G, Chappel CI, Kahn DS. The significance of factors modifying the development of isoproterenol induced myocardial necrosis. *Am Heart J* 1963; **66**: 389–95.
25. Symons C. Altered thyroid function and cardiac disease. In: Bristow MR, ed. *Drug-induced heart disease*. Amsterdam: Biomedical Press, 1980; 421–31.
26. Bristow MR, Ginsburg R, Harrison DC. Histamine and the human heart: the other receptor system. *Am J Cardiol* 1982; **49**: 249–51.
27. Ginsburg R, Bristow MR, Harrison DC, Stinson EB. Studies with isolated human coronary arteries. Some general observations, potential mediators of spasm, role of calcium antagonists. *Chest* 1980; **78**: 180S–6S.
28. Adelstein RS, Hathaway DR. Role of calcium and cyclic adenosine 3′:5′ monophosphate in regulating smooth muscle contraction. Mechanisms of excitation–contraction coupling in smooth muscle. *Am J Cardiol* 1979; **44**: 783–7.
29. Mackay D. A new method for the analysis of drug-receptor interactions. *Adv Drug Res* 1966; **3**: 1–19.
30. McConnaughey MM, Jones LR, Watanabe AM et al. Thyroxine and propylthiourcil effects on alpha- and beta-adrenergic receptor number, ATPase activities, and sialic acid content of rat cardiac membrane vesicles. *J Cardiovasc Pharm* 1979; **1**: 609–23.
31. Smitherman RC, Johnson RS, Taubert K et al. Acute thyrotoxicosis in the rabbit: changes in cardiac myosin, contractility, and ultra-structure. *Biochem Med* 1979; **21**: 277–98.
32. Lewis SJ, Luric K, Bristow MR, Sageman WS, Ginsburg R, Billingham ME. Myocardial β-adrenergic receptor up-regulation in rabbits fed a high cholesterol diet. (Abstract). *Circulation*, 1981; **64** (Suppl. 4): iv–207.
33. Lurie K, Bristow M, Ginsburg R et al. Vascular H_1-receptor up-regulation in rabbits fed a high cholesterol diet. (Abstract.) *Circulation*, 1981; **64** (Suppl. 4): iv–272.
34. Bristow MR, Ginsburg R, Sageman WS, Billingham ME, Stinson EB. Analysis of the beta-adrenergic receptor pathway in myocardial disease. (Abstract.) *Circulation*, 1981; **64** (Suppl. 4): iv–286.
35. Bristow MR, ed. *Drug-induced heart disease*. Amsterdam: Biomedical Press, 1980.

Chapter 11

Diseases of the transplanted heart

Margaret E. Billingham

INTRODUCTION

This chapter will review the current survival rates in cardiac transplantation, and some of the homograft pathology affecting survival in long-term cardiac recipients. The data for this study are from Stanford University Hospital Clinical Cardiac Transplant Programme, which is now in its thirteenth year. In this programme 227 cardiac transplants have been performed on 206 patients with ages ranging from 12 to 55 years. Nineteen patients have been retransplanted for the first time (2 for immediate graft failure, 5 for relentless acute rejection and 12 for graft atherosclerosis), and 2 patients have been retransplanted for the second time for early graft failure and graft atherosclerosis. The total number of patients surviving 1 year is 107, and there are 75 long-term survivors, up to 11 years following cardiac transplant. Eighty per cent of the recipients are rehabilitated, the definition of rehabilitation being that they have returned to at least American Heart Association Class 1 functional ability; many of them have gone back to college, their professions or jobs. In 1974 the clinical management of cardiac recipients was improved by the use of the endomyocardial biopsy and the use of rabbit antithymocyte globulin which improved the survival statistics. *Figure 1* shows the overall survival figures as well as the improved figures after 1974. The main attrition is in the first 3 months following transplantation. At 1 year there is over 62 per cent survival, and there is a 42 per cent survival at 5 years. From this group there are patients in the 6, 7, 8, 9, 10 and 11 year survival range. A 50 per cent survival rate at 5 years might not be considered good for most diseases, but attention should be drawn to the fact that those patients accepted (by the rather rigorous criteria) for cardiac transplantation at Stanford

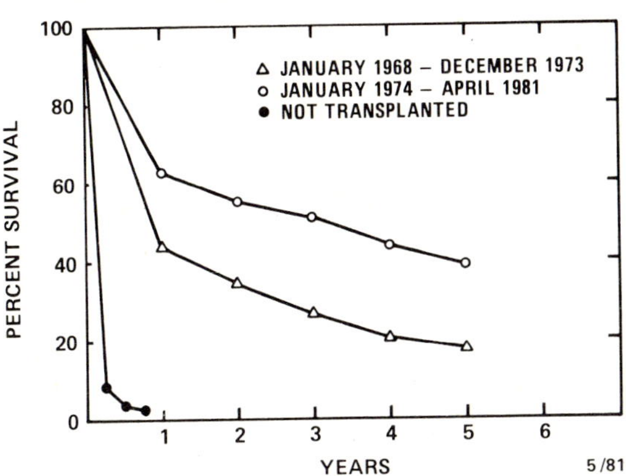

Figure 1. Graph of survival statistics for the Stanford University Medical School Cardiac Transplant Programme in humans.

have an average lifespan of only 55 days if a suitable donor does not become available. There is a special group which enjoys a slightly higher survival rate: this is a group of cardiac recipients who have had previous cardiac surgery for cardiac valve replacement, aneurysmectomy or coronary artery bypass operation. These patients have a slightly higher 1 year survival rate of 68 per cent. In addition, there is a higher survival rate in those patients who have been transplanted in the past 3 years, and those who are younger than 20 years at operation.

The causes of death in the 110 cardiac transplant recipients who did not survive are shown in Table 1. It can be seen that a very large

Table 1
Stanford cardiac transplantation

Primary cause of death		
Infection	76/131	58%
Acute rejection	23/131	17·5%
Pulmonary hypertension	5/131	3·9%
Graft arteriosclerosis		
(a) Proliferative	5/131	3·8%
(b) Atherosclerotic	9/131	6·9%
Malignancy	6/131	4·6%
CVA	3/131	4·6%
Suicide	1/131	0·8%
Pulmonary embolus	2/131	1·5%
Unknown	1/131	0·8%

number of recipient deaths are due to infection,[1–4] primarily of the lungs but also septicaemia, urinary tract, disseminated fungal, central nervous system, hepatitis, retinitis and miscellaneous infections, as are seen in other immunosuppressed patient populations. Acute rejection, usually manifested in the first 3 months after transplantation, is the next highest cause of death. Graft atherosclerosis, both proliferative and atherosclerotic, accounts for the highest proportion of deaths in long-term survivors. In our series 4·6 per cent of cardiac recipients have succumbed to malignancies, mainly undifferentiated lymphomas.[5] Pulmonary hypertension, occasionally occurring in patients who have had chronic cardiac disease for some time prior to transplantation, causes difficulty immediately after transplantation as the new, unhypertrophied right ventricle cannot support the high pulmonary vascular resistance. This predicament can now be alleviated by a combined heart–lung transplantation which has been performed successfully on two occasions at Stanford. The remaining deaths were caused by cerebrovascular accident, suicide and pulmonary embolus.

PROBLEMS FOLLOWING HEART TRANSPLANTATION

Infection

From Table 1 it can be seen that the highest cause of death in cardiac transplant recipients is from infections due to the massive immunosuppression that they receive. The infection is usually systemic, most often pulmonary and may include bacterial, viral, fungal, rickettsial and other unusual opportunistic organisms. This aspect will not be dealt with in detail here since infection of the myocardium itself is not usually a cause of heart failure in this group of patients. When there is disseminated fungal infection the donor heart may of course be affected. There have been several cases of disseminated toxoplasmosis in which the heart has been involved. By use of routine endomyocardial biopsies of postoperative patients, these infections are occasionally diagnosed from the biopsy material (*Figure 2*). At Stanford, toxoplasmosis, cytomegalic viral inclusions and coccidioidomycosis have been picked up unexpectedly on a routine endomyocardial biopsy.

Allograft Rejection

It can be seen from Table 1 that acute allograft rejection in both the acute and chronic forms remains the single most challenging problem in effecting successful cardiac transplantation in man. At Stanford, cardiac recipients and donors are matched only for ABO blood groups, absence of cytotoxic effects of the recipient serum to the donor leucocytes, and although histocompatibility tests are performed on all

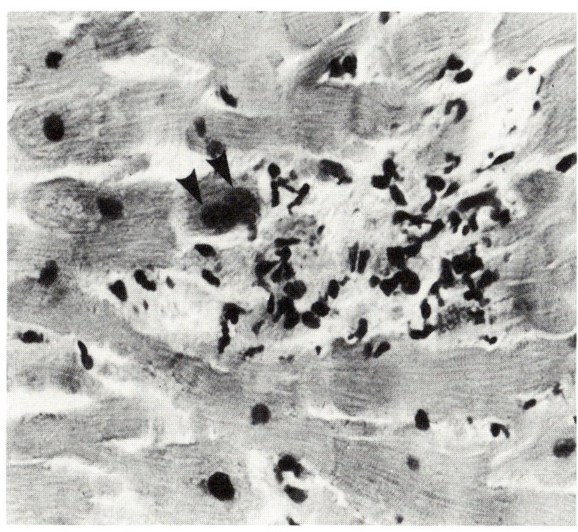

Figure 2. Photomicrograph from endomyocardial biopsy showing cyst of Toxoplasma gondii.

patients and because of the small number of available donors, this is not usually used for prospective matching.

The gross appearance of the donor heart in end stage acute rejection is large, swollen, very firm from interstitial oedema, with swelling and turgidity of the intraventricular trabeculae, the papillary muscles, and sometimes of the valves. The endocardial and cut surfaces show patchy haemorrhage which imparts a dark plum-coloured hue to the myocardium. There is often a marked contrast of myocardial texture and colour along the atrial suture lines between the recipient and donor hearts in acute rejection.

In order to diagnose acute rejection at its onset the endomyocardial biopsy is performed routinely on all cardiac transplant recipients. Several methods for human heart biopsy with a catheter bioptome have been developed and reported in the literature.[6–11] At Stanford the percutaneous transvenous method developed by Caves et al. is used.[12–15] This method is rapid, can be frequently repeated and is well tolerated by the patients (one cardiac recipient had 38 endomyocardial biopsies). In order to reduce sampling error, at each biopsy procedure 3–5 small pieces of myocardium (2–3 mm in maximum dimension) are obtained from the interventricular septum. At Stanford, where over 3000 endomyocardial biopsies have been performed, there have been no deaths as a result of the procedure and morbidity has been less than 1 per cent.

Over 2000 endomyocardial biopsies have been performed on 206 cardiac recipients at Stanford. This experience has provided the basis for the definition and grading of the histopathological changes in acute cardiac rejection.[16]

Early Acute Rejection

This is amenable to treatment and is easily reversible. There is interstitial and sometimes endocardial oedema and, concomitantly, a scanty and predominantly perivascular infiltrate of immunoblasts (immunologically stimulated lymphocytes) which are pyroninophilic (*Figure 3A*). At this stage endothelial cells of the endocardium and small vessels are also pyroninophilic.

Moderate Acute Rejection

A moderate acute rejection can also be reversed relatively easily with augmented immunosuppression. At this stage the inflammatory infiltrate of immunoblasts is increased and is more diffuse throughout the interstitium (*Figure 3B*). Early, focal myocyte necrosis may be seen—this can be highlighted by the use of a Masson's trichrome stain.

Severe Acute Rejection

This is usually not reversible. The inflammatory infiltrate now includes neutrophils, there is interstitial and perivascular haemorrhage, and vascular and myocyte necrosis (*Figure 3C*).

Resolving Acute Rejection

If the rejection process is reversed by therapy the biopsy will show active fibrosis, haemosiderin deposits and a residual infiltrate of small (non-pyroninophilic) lymphocytes and plasma cells (*Figure 3D*).

The inflammatory infiltrate of mononuclear cells in acute cellular rejection has been shown in earlier animal studies to be T cells.[17] More recently, with the development of human T cell antibodies, the infiltrate in human rejection has been shown to contain all the T cell subgroups, varying in amount with the immunosuppression used (unpublished data).

Immunofluorescence can be used on the frozen pieces of the endomyocardial biopsies. In acute rejection, immunoglobulin deposition in the myocardium can be seen; however, this is modified by the treatment. In our hands this method has been non-predictive and unreliable for the management of acute rejection.

Transvenous endomyocardial biopsy provides an accurate, objective

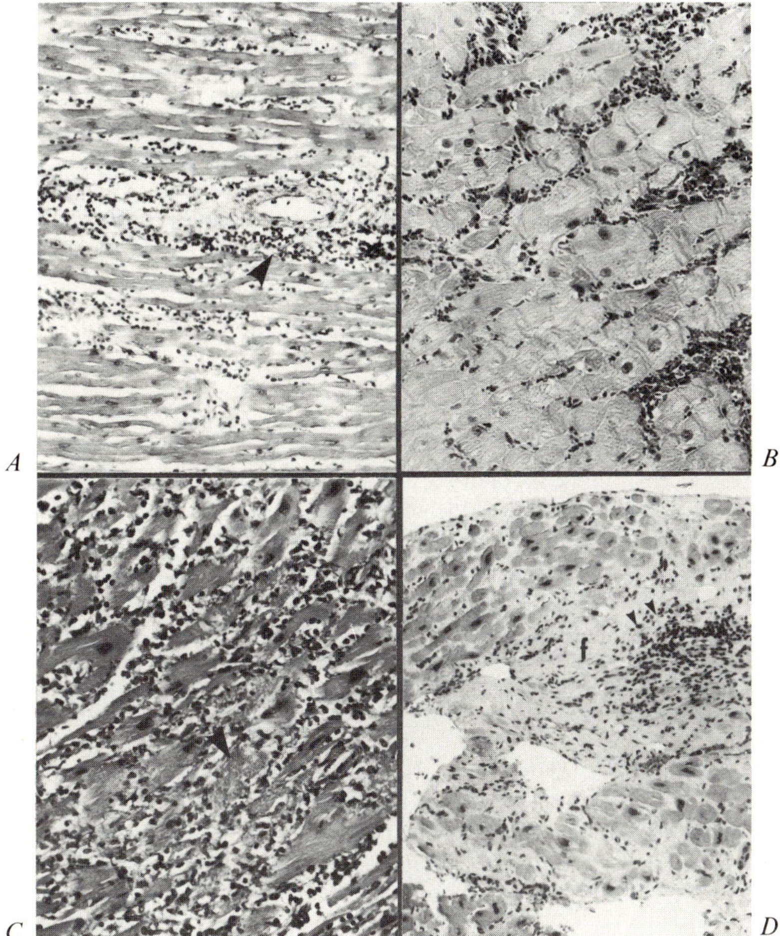

Figure 3. (A) Mild acute rejection in a biopsy showing interstitial oedema and perivascular (arrow) mononuclear infiltrate. (B) Moderate acute rejection: increase in interstitial mononuclear infiltrate. (C) Severe acute rejection: increased mixed inflammatory infiltrate with myocyte necrosis (arrow). (D) Resolving acute rejection: note the fibrosis (f) and residual small lymphocytes (arrow) in the scar.

histological evaluation of graft status which has evolved into an important part of the clinical management in cardiac recipients. Its use has allowed effective early treatment of a rejection process and it has also prevented unnecessary augmentation of immunosuppressive therapy.

Graft Atherosclerosis

As can be seen from Table 1, graft atherosclerosis, either proliferative or atherosclerotic, accounts for 14 of 131 deaths of cardiac recipients and has accounted for 13 of 21 retransplantation procedures undertaken at Stanford. In general, atherosclerosis of major coronary arteries following cardiac transplantation is histopathologically similar to that occurring in the natural state. Although focal stenotic lesions can and do occur, in general the coronary vessels tend to be affected throughout their length, which is in keeping with the theory of immunological insult to the vascular endothelium. In a critical examination of our series of cardiac transplant survivors we have not been able to attach a clear-cut causal relationship between accelerated atherosclerosis and the number of rejection episodes, previous heart disease (coronary or cardiomyopathy), histocompatibility matching, sex of the donor or recipient, or treatment regimen. The length of time from transplant also does not appear to be related. The appearance of atherosclerosis in the coronary arteries has been substantially mitigated with close attention to weight control, diet, antiplatelet aggregating agents and keeping serum lipoproteins to a low or normal level.[18] All cardiac transplant survivors have annual coronary arteriograms to monitor the onset of coronary vascular disease.

The proliferative type of coronary vascular disease is much more insidious, particularly when it affects only the smaller penetrating coronary artery branches. This type of proliferation may occur early and will not necessarily show up on the coronary arteriograms although a 'slow flow' phenomenon may be picked up by an astute radiologist. We have had a cardiac recipient die suddenly 1 year after transplantation, and 1 month after an apparently normal coronary arteriogram, of a massive myocardial infarction due to 'small vessel disease'. At autopsy all the penetrating branches of the coronary arteries were partially or totally occluded by intimal proliferation (*Figure 4*). The policy now at Stanford is to retransplant those patients with known coronary artery disease as sudden death may ensue.

DONOR HEART PRESERVATION FOR CARDIAC TRANSPLANTATION

The paucity of donor hearts available for human transplantation can be remedied by distant heart procurement. The main difference in technique between on-site heart procurement and distant heart procurement is the use of a cardioplegic solution for metabolic arrest and cooling of the heart in the latter situation. This technique is described in greater detail elsewhere.[19,20] After the heart is excised, it is placed in a sterile bag and a sterile, saline-filled cannister which is packed in ice

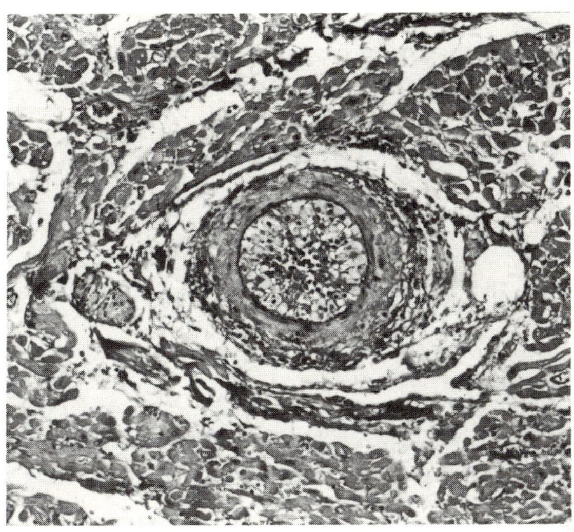

Figure 4. Transverse section of a small intramyocardial artery showing marked intimal proliferation in a cardiac allograft 1 year after transplantation.

for transport. At Stanford, hearts with a maximum of 3 hours' ischaemic time have been transplanted successfully with up to 3 years' survival so far.[21]

Ultrastructural changes seen at a mean ischaemic time of 154 minutes (transported hearts) were minimal when compared with the changes seen in on-site donors with a mean 49 minute ischaemic time, with the exception of changes in the vascular endothelium. The capillary endothelium was intact, without blebs or swelling in the on-site donors, whereas it was damaged in all of the distantly obtained hearts. Ultrastructural examination, obtained by endomyocardial biopsies taken 30 minutes after transplantation and reperfusion, showed an increase in degenerative changes with nuclear chromatin clumping and margination, mitochondrial swelling, myocyte contraction bands, focal cell necrosis, platelet aggregation and endothelial damage. After reperfusion there was capillary damage seen from the biopsies of the on-site donors as well. Survival of the recipients who received transported hearts in this study is 63 per cent $\pm$ 8 per cent compared with 55 per cent $\pm$ 4 per cent for recipients who received on-site donor hearts. In our studies we could not distinguish any ultrastructural changes in one group from those of the other 1 year later. Rehabilitation and exercise tolerance did not differ between the two groups. These studies suggest that a simple preservation technique can be used to preserve donor hearts for at least 3 hours with satisfactory function and survival of the recipient. All the morphological changes described appear to be reversible. The limits of ischaemia for this form of preservation are not yet established.

MORPHOLOGICAL STUDIES ON LONG-TERM SURVIVORS OF CARDIAC TRANSPLANTATION

Endomyocardial biopsies on long-term survivors of heart transplants from 1 to 8 years show cardiac morphology which is within normal limits. There is usually a definite increase in interstitial fibrosis from normal and occasionally there are residual aggregates of non-pyroninophilic lymphocytes. Likewise electron microscopic examination of endomyocardial biopsies show areas that are quite indistinguishable from normal myocardium, including the interstitium. The number of nerve endings is much fewer than in normal myocardium because the heart is denervated at transplantation. Normal nerve endings which presumably are residual post-ganglionic parasympathetic fibres can be seen, some containing dense core granules. There is no evidence that reinnervation of the heart takes place at this time. Electrophysiological studies including challenging the donor heart with atropine, tyramine and amyl nitrate have failed to show physiological reinnervation as of 8 years' post-cardiac transplantation.

Accelerated atherosclerosis in the donor hearts of long-term cardiac allograft survivors has been alluded to earlier in this chapter. Our experience at Stanford suggests that at 5 years post-transplant, 38 per cent of the donor hearts will have some disease of the coronary arteries.

I would like to conclude this review of disease in the transplanted heart by suggesting that cardiac transplantation really does constitute a genuine therapeutic alternative for highly selected and carefully managed patients. The survival rates for cardiac allografts are comparable or even superior to those reported for renal transplants in unrelated donors. The quality of life achieved by 80 per cent of the cardiac recipients is much improved.

REFERENCES

1. Stinson EB, Bieber CP, Griepp RB, Clark DA, Shumway NE, and Remington JS. Infectious complications after cardiac transplantation in man. *Ann Intern Med* 1971; **74**: 22.
2. Remington JS, Gaines DJ, Griepp RB, Shumway NE. Further experience with infection after cardiac transplantation. *Transplant Proc* 1972; **4**: 699.
3. Rand KH, Rasmussen LE, Pollard RB, Arvin A, Merigan TC. Cellular immunity and herpes virus infections in cardiac transplant patients. *N Engl J Med* 1976; **296**: 1372.

4. Schober R, Herman M. Neuropathology of cardiac transplantation—a survey of 31 cases. *Lancet* 1973; **1**: 962.
5. Krikorian JG, Anderson JL, Bieber CP, Penn I, Stinson E. Malignant neoplasms following cardiac transplantation. *JAMA* 1978; **240**: 639.
6. Sakakibara S, Konno S. Endomyocardial biopsy. *Jap Heart J* 1962; **3**: 537.
7. Konno S, Sakakibara S. Endomyocardial biopsy. *Dis Chest* 1963; **44**: 345.
8. Sakakibara S, Konno S. Intracardiac heart biopsy. *Jap Circ J* 1966; **30**: 1582.
9. Ali N. Transvenous endomyocardial biopsy using the gastrointestinal biopsy (Olympus GFB) catheter. *Am Heart J* 1974; **87**: 294.
10. Richardson PJ. King's endomyocardial bioptome. *Lancet* 1974; **1**: 660.
11. Brooksky IAB *et al.* Left ventricular endomyocardial biopsy. *Lancet* 1974; **2**: 1222.
12. Caves PK, Schulz WP, Dong E Jr et al. A new instrument for transvenous cardiac biopsy. *Am J Cardiol* 1974; **33**: 264.
13. Caves PK, Stinson EB, Billingham ME, Shumway NE. Transvenous intracardiac biopsy using a new catheter forceps. *Heart Lung* 1975; **4**: 69.
14. Caves PK, Stinson EB, Graham AF, Billingham ME, Grehl TM, Shumway NE. Percutaneous transvenous endomyocardial biopsy. *JAMA* 1973; **225**: 289.
15. Caves PK, Stinson EB, Billingham ME et al. Percutaneous transvenous endomyocardial biopsy in human heart recipients (experience with a new technique). *Ann Thor Surg* 1973; **3**: 117.
16. Billingham ME. Some recent advances in cardiac pathology. *Hum Pathol* 1979; **10**: 367.
17. Billingham M, Warnke R, Weissman I. The cellular infiltrate in cardiac allograft rejection in mice. *Transplantation* 1977; **23**: 171–6.
18. Griepp RB, Stinson EB, Bieber CP et al. Control of graft arteriosclerosis in human heart transplant recipients. *Surgery* 1977; **81**: 262.
19. Stinson EB, Dong ED Jr, Iben AB, Shumway NE. Cardiac transplantation in man—surgical aspects. *Am J Surg* 1969; **118**: 182.
20. Reitz BA, Stinson EB. *Profound local hypothermia for myocardial protection.* Presented at the Symposium on Intraoperative Myocardial Protection, Cologne, Germany, October 2–4, 1979.
21. Billingham ME, Baumgartner MD, Watson DC et al. Distant heart procurement for human transplantation. *Circulation* 1980; **62**: suppl. 1: 1–11.

Index